THE POSTPARTUM PATH OF YOGA

The Postpartum Path of Yoga

A Program for Restoration of Body, Mind, Voice, & Spirit

MELISSA HURT

Integrative Studio

DEDICATION

*I dedicate this book
to my daughter,
Penny, whose birth
and first years
brought me to the
edges of extreme
living and whose love
and grace inspired me
to re-capture my best
self to give her the
mother she deserves.*

CONTENTS

~ 1 ~

INTRODUCTION

I lay on the examination table in my midwife's office in shock. I was 29 weeks pregnant and found out my daughter was breech. If she did not flip to a head-down position, I'd have to have a C-section.

I felt stunned and, honestly, a little betrayed. I did everything the midwife prescribed for a healthy pregnancy: I ate a whole foods diet (no bread! no baked goods!), drank tons of water, taught yoga three times a week, and practiced yoga almost daily. Despite all my work, the doctors had to subject me to an operation, denying me the opportunity to have a natural, vaginal birth for which I had hoped and planned. I didn't have the final say in how things went because another living being who also had a say was involved. *My first lesson in parenting:* **It is a collaboration, a relationship.**

I was scared of many things: The C-section itself, complications from the surgery, the effect on my baby, having a difficult recovery, to name a few. On the day of the operation, I waited five hours from when I arrived at the hospital to the beginning of the surgery. I received the epidural, the dividing sheet went up, the ob/gyn made the incision, and, within ten minutes, the assisting medical students pushed the baby downward. I felt a wave-like motion from my breathing diaphragm all the way to my pelvis. The doctor proclaimed, "Oh! She's beautiful, you guys!"

My daughter took her first breath and then cried. The sound of her voice brought me to tears—no, not tears but sobs. So miraculous! All the pain, trials, discomfort, and morning sickness I'd been through had disappeared. I was now enveloped in the glory of motherhood. I felt so blessed, so fortunate to hear those adorable baby cries, and so certain that my role in life was to be the best mother I could possibly be for that little girl.

The glory came with hardship. My time in the hospital following surgery was treacherous. No one told me about the vacuum effect that can happen once air seeps inside an open abdomen. When the doctor sutured me, air stayed inside me and created immense pressure and pain in my abdomen—an intensity of pain I'd never felt before.

Ironically, the nurses advised me to walk around the hospital floor to relieve the gas and pressure. Yet, I was in so much pain I could hardly move. How could I walk an entire hospital floor if I couldn't stand upright? Next came the continual wake-ups to nurse my daughter through the night. I didn't mind at first, but after the first month of navigating new motherhood at home, the feedings took a massive toll on my energy. Previously, I had no idea how crazy sleep deprivation can make a person.

Add to that the restrictions to my diet. I hoped I could relax a bit from the whole foods, the non-processed-food diet I'd endured throughout my pregnancy. But after Penny's birth, I had to be extra vigilant not to eat beans or cruciferous vegetables (broccoli, cabbage, cauliflower) because I had heard they'd make my daughter gassy. Plus, constantly nursing her made me feel like I was starving all the time.

My family visited over the first three weeks. Once they left, my husband returned to work, leaving me home alone with our daughter. This email message sent by a friend became my *mantra* during this time: "Her self-esteem is yours to nurture or destroy."

Wow. That means it's my job to create the neurological wiring for her sense of self that sets her up in the world for the rest of her life. *Right,* I thought, *I can do this: I totally understand her and know what she needs.* It was the pep talk I gave myself every morning after my husband shut the door, not to return for eight hours or more.

I knew I needed to give her my best, with the only way being to *find* my best.

But the isolation led me to depression. The sleep deprivation made me feel delirious and unable to safely drive a car, especially maneuvering in parking garages with all the lines and columns. I saw a therapist weekly, bringing my daughter with me. The therapist helped me understand how isolating motherhood can be in contemporary society. I felt better knowing I'm not alone in my loneliness.

Then One Day, It Happened...

I was exhausted. I had just put my baby in the crib for a nap. I prayed she'd sleep more than 20 minutes so I could talk on the phone with Nancy, my dear friend and embodied voice certification mentor. We chatted for a few minutes before she called me out on this: *I had little to no vocal tone or vibrancy to my voice.* How could I, a certified trainer of our work, speak that way?

Nancy asked if I read stories to my daughter. "Yes, all the time," I replied. She suggested that *feeling* my voice would be a healthy way to regain my vocal life and find a new way to connect with my daughter. I knew how. *My second lesson in parenting:* **I couldn't give my daughter my best if I weren't taking care of myself.**

From that moment on, I took pleasure in playing with my voice while I read. I noticed how I felt my voice as I spoke while also sustaining a connection to my body and my surroundings. As my body recovered, I could dance with my baby and enjoy balance and rhythm as a part of my physical and spiritual healing. I was getting back my health and emotional wellness while inadvertently discovering how paying attention to my voice and body was an act of mindfulness.

That's when I made a point of going on stroller walks in the morning and afternoon. That's when I made 4:00 p.m. my music hour and loudly played songs from my adolescence as I danced with my daughter. As she got older, we played with toy musical instruments. Honestly, having a schedule was the only way to hold onto some everyday life.

Eventually, I joined a playgroup of theatre parents in the Washington, DC area. There I met people who would become my closest friends. My daughter could grow up with babies who would become her best friends. One day, I met a mom in my neighborhood on a stroller walk, and she became a very close friend of mine. Years later, she would be my go-to friend for girls' night out. This small community of friends saved me over the years from babyhood to preschooler. I met them by consciously deciding to put on daytime clothes, leave the house, and work on being social. What started as a chore became pleasurable.

The whole of my professional work—as a certified yoga teacher and embodied voice and movement trainer—gave me the tools I needed to get my life back on track. It's having the wisdom to connect with a community that further lifted me out of the dregs. I didn't want my daughter to grow up with an exhausted, burned-out mommy. Deep in my soul, I knew she deserved a mother who felt well so I could take good care of her. She deserved the best of me. I did, too.

My path to restoration had begun.

It had taken five months of exhaustion to fry my voice. It had taken two and half years to become so anxious and mentally depleted that I had little patience for daily life. It took four years of moving before I developed pelvic pain and pelvic floor imbalances due to a lack of understanding about the core and the pelvic floor. To rehabilitate, I turned to embodied voice practices, meditation, and an astute education of the core and movement. I have used all I have learned and experienced as a launching pad for intensive study and devotion to postnatal recovery and wellness. As a result, I have created this program for you.

Everything You Need Is Within...

When my daughter was three years old, I came across Parker J. Palmer's work at a time I felt more solidly rooted in my life. He wrote in *Let Your Life Speak*: "'Seasons' is a wise metaphor for the movement of life, I think . . . The notion that our lives are like the eternal cycle of the seasons does not deny the struggle or the joy, the loss or the gain, the darkness or the light, but encourages us to embrace it all—and to find in all of it the opportunities for growth."[1]

I often reflect on Palmer's analogy of "life in seasons" when I witness the span of experiences among the mothers I teach in my yoga classes. Some have babies that refuse sleep; some have babies that struggle to nurse or take a bottle without reflux; others have babies that do both so beautifully that their mothers feel guilty about how they got so lucky. Mothers of older children share stories of how they balance being a teacher of life skills, a protector, and an observer of their child's struggle to figure things out independently. It's a constant battle with a mother's energy.

Consistently, though, mothers encounter a range of temperaments and trials with their children. I recall this beloved lyric in Fleetwood Mac's song Landslide: "Can I handle the seasons of my life?" Although it's helpful to find life occurring in seasons because it promises that "this, too, shall pass," sometimes we don't know if we can handle the tumult of sleep deprivation, lack of community support, and/or stress. Can I get through this phase? I often embraced singer Stevie Nicks' answer: "I don't know."[2]

But now, I can tell you this: "Yes, you can." You have everything you need inside of you to get through the darkest days of motherhood, whether you have a baby or a spirited older child. And you can seek community support once you tap into your inner-felt resources to get well. From all my years working with new mothers, I think of the abrupt changes a new baby brings as winter. Even when your days are busy, your baby is beautiful, and it seems like springtime, at the essence, is a stillness and quiet that presents growth potential. Palmer shared, "Winter clears the landscape, however brutally, giving us a chance to see ourselves and each other more clearly, to see the very ground of our being."[3] Just as the ground is barren on a snowless day in winter, we can choose to see the foundation of ourselves if we have the courage and stillness to look inward. This is the time to rest whenever possible and foster as much self-care as possible while caring for your baby. Conserve your energy in the fourth trimester—your baby's first three months —so you have resources to sustain yourself once the baby is more mobile. Over time, your energy steadies, and your spirit focuses on your deeply felt values for self-care and family care.

Winter will come again as your child ages, and your relationship takes on new dynamics. Your task is to explore when you press on your values to teach or protect your child and when you hold back and trust they can use the tools you have taught them so far to navigate a situation. Sometimes sitting in the shadows means letting your child take the light and lead. Your child may be able to teach you something at this time of winter. You will find replenishment and inspiration again and feel the vitality of spring when you enter the next phase of your relationship, which further shapes your identity as a mother.

The choices we make today affect what comes later. When a mother takes care of herself, she sustains herself and the baby beyond the fourth trimester into their adventure ahead. The mothers I work with ride the tide and eventually find their way onto steady ground. Amid the ups and downs of motherhood, their quest for the light of personal growth at the center of darkness is a beautiful and worthy endeavor. It's a path that's treacherous, inspiring, and wonderful all at once. And it starts as soon as a mother sets the intention to practice wellness day in and day out.

Remember, your intention is a promise to yourself that nurtures your soul. It's what you work toward cultivating every time you open this book and commit to this program week after week. The moment Nancy challenged me to connect with my essential self every time I spoke, I intended to become the most vital woman I could be—for myself and my family.

I am a certified yoga teacher and certified embodied voice, speech, and movement trainer. Through the mothers I've met in postnatal yoga classes (with babies and toddlers), I have encountered as much fear, frustration, and anxiety about motherhood as I have witnessed bliss and joy—to the point of beautiful tears coming to my eyes. Older mothers share stories proving this range of emotions remains as they nurture their children into adulthood.

For all the resources on the market on prenatal care and the birthing process, a mother is typically left in the dark about how to take care of herself now that she has a new baby. A multitude of books offer solutions on how to take care of a baby. They range in topics from sleep training to breastfeeding to diapering to baby-led weaning and feeding solid foods. These books help thousands of mothers choose which actions best support their baby's health and development. But there are fewer books on the market that teach mothers how to take care of themselves, especially regarding body, mind, voice, and spirit.

The Postpartum Path of Yoga answers the silent scream women emote once they have given birth. There is a void in knowing how to take care of herself through ways that acknowledge changes in her body (physiological and anatomical), her unpredictable emotions, and her relationship with herself and others. She wants to feel balanced, present, and well once again. I consider this lack of information a crisis in women's health. We shall no longer feel confused and ashamed by how we feel upon entering motherhood while devoting ourselves to taking care of a child. Let's be honest with our experiences and find strategies to cope and grow, so we feel better and stronger in body, mind, voice, and spirit in the process and on the other side of confusion, fatigue, and anxiety.

The Postpartum Path of Yoga instructs you on how to connect with yourself over your first year of motherhood and beyond. It offers a five-pronged program of breath-based practices, yoga and other mindful movements, embodied voice exploration, meditation, and a study of the ethical guidelines and observances in yoga called the *yamas* and *niyamas*. This book is for all mothers, regardless of their child's age and the number of children they have had. The information and practices are suitable once a doctor has cleared you for an exercise/movement program. This typically occurs between six and eight weeks after giving birth, depending on whether you've had a vaginal birth or a C-section. The movement practice is appropriate for women completely new to yoga postures and those experienced in yoga.

I recommend creating a discipline by doing the program six days a week, with the seventh being a day of rest and community building. However, I fully understand how different one day is from the next based on the sleep you and the baby get, schedule changes, a work/family balance struggle, and the unpredictability of daily life despite your best efforts to create a routine.

If you can only devote four days a week to the program, feel content with that and work toward a six-day commitment as you find your stride. I recommend that mothers of babies find ways to do the program when their baby naps or is happily playing with toys nearby. You can do the practices sequentially or one at a time as you move through the day if you are time-constrained.

You'll find at the heart of your study with me is a lesson from the *Yoga Sutras*, the classical text teaching the practice and art of yoga. This self-development practice brings you to an integration of the heart-mind with the Divine energy that surrounds us. The integration leads to what's called *samadhi*, or true bliss. *Yoga Sutras* 1.20 and 1.21 state: "For most people, (deep insight into complete absorption of the heart-mind) is preceded by faith, vitality, strong memory, samadhi, then deep insight. Intense momentum of practice and faith accelerates them toward samadhi."[4]

There it is: **The first step in the practice of self-betterment is faith.**

If you don't have faith that this path will take you somewhere, why create the discipline to do it at all? The best approach is to practice for the *enjoyment of the practice* and the time you're spending with yourself—enjoy the sensations of what you feel and do and the boost in energy that comes during and after practice.

Those who commit to a path attached to a perceived result usually end up frustrated and not completing the program. Why? Because they aren't spiritually invested in *the thing itself.* They are only committed to a result on an ego level. Instead, I invite you to practice for the sake of practice and discovery. Work to detach from the fruits of your work each day to start the next day anew and enjoy the work as it comes moment by moment.

Once we find faith in what we do, we can practice with vitality. There must be a spark of commitment, love, and devotion in our actions that feels vital. Otherwise, we are empty shells going through the motions. Then we want to have strong, sustained memories so our minds focus on what we do and feel. We're tapped into the inner light within. Next, we find *samadhi*—blissful and complete absorption/integration with the inner light. Last, we have deep insights about ourselves from moving through these stages.

This is the journey *The Postpartum Path of Yoga* extends to you. It is up to you to see it through. Make an intention every day you practice that brings you back to *why* you are committed to self-development. What do you hope to create within that helps you connect more deeply with the world? What brings you back day after day? Let your answer speak to your values and deep-felt connections to yourself. This will be the flickering light deep in your soul that shines on the path ahead. The momentum of your practice will further lead you to your bliss as the work becomes a way of life.

Let your answer speak to your values and deep-felt connections to yourself. This will be the flickering light deep in your soul that shines on the path ahead.

How This Program Is Organized

The program featured in *The Postpartum Path of Yoga* is set up in four parts. **Part One** starts the path toward healing by illustrating common physiological and anatomical circumstances experienced by many women after having a baby that can last for years. This gives you a foundation on which to build your wellness practice. I call it "The Five Conditions You Don't Have to Accept" because it lays out five common ailments of postnatal life that tend to affect women for years. The physiological and anatomical components of each condition are explained so you can understand how they correlate.

PART ONE

Part One explains the current research on postnatal depletion; the neuroscience of isolation, which many women feel after having a baby; the effect cortisol (the fight-flight-or-freeze hormone) has on the body when women are sleep deprived, anxious, and lack optimal nutrition; and the causes of vocal fry and vocal fatigue that rob their spiritual energy.

You'll read about the anatomy of the female pelvis and the torso making up the core, including the pelvic floor. Knowing this grounds your movement-based practices in understanding the body's architecture and how its parts work best as an *integrated system* that shares the workload through your body. You allow the particulars of this anatomical material to inform you of the complexity of *you* and guide your understanding of movement-based practices.

You'll read about the anatomical groundwork for the crux of your breath and movement-based work. It discusses balancing the pelvic floor, healing the separation of the abdominal sheath in the front of the body (commonly known as "diastasis recti"), and toning the whole of the core from the inside out.

Why include lessons in physiology and anatomy? It's so you can understand how and why your body and mind differ from what you may have experienced pre-pregnancy. The ligaments of the pelvis have taken on strain to carry the load of pregnancy and deliver a baby. Multiple pregnancies weaken the ligaments further. Your movement practices work to preserve the pelvis's integrity as it heals. You will focus on safely developing core strength that can support the pelvis as you move, and you'll learn to move your pelvis in ways that keep its two halves stable. This pelvis alignment heals as you strengthen and stabilize surrounding muscles.

New mothers ought not to plunge back into physical practices they did before having their baby. This can feel confusing since they think they *should* be the same person with a beautiful addition to the family. If they loved running and high-intensity interval training (known as HIIT) pre-pregnancy, why can't they start up again once they are cleared for movement by their doctors or midwives? Mothers are not in the physical condition they were in before growing, carrying, and birthing a child. Instead, they require a modified physical practice to get to know themselves intimately. Mothers need to investigate ranges of motion as they begin moving again. This helps them recover from childbearing and rebuild their bodies appropriately and safely. Adding a baby isn't like acquiring a family pet. Mothers need time to adapt to the changes in their schedules, sleep, nutrition, and physicality.

As a new mom, your body, mind, and spirit are in transition. *The Postpartum Path of Yoga* will give you the tools to feel grounded throughout the evolution. I recommend exploring the movement-based practices at a slow yet focused, pace over the first year as you learn to respect how your body heals. You can repeat the program as often as you can through the first year postpartum. I hope you find compassion for yourself along the way and continue learning more and more about yourself.

PART TWO

Part Two launches the program over six phases through:

- a regimen of breath-based practices;
- movements from the yoga tradition and other traditions;
- embodied voice and speech explorations; and
- meditations.

You'll learn about the yoga modifications you need and why you won't find lunges and planks in **Part Two** of this program. I recommend practicing at least four to (as many as) six days a week, with the seventh day being a rest day.

You'll see how I break down each phase into weeks that incrementally feed into each successive phase. Over the course of the program, you'll feel like you know yourself better and can reclaim your bodymind (i.e., the integration of body, mind, memory, emotion, and intelligence that is you) as home to your spirit. Every time you look within, I hope you will feel like you're entering a safe space where you can simply *be.*

Each phase begins with a prompt for finding a community. This gives you ideas about getting social and finding your "mama tribe." If you don't have an immediate support network, you can create one, and I offer suggestions for how to do this.

Each day, you will start with a breath-based centering practice to connect mind, body, breath, and spirit. From here, you'll learn movement-based practices mostly (from the yogic tradition) to get to know your body as it is today and work toward improving your strength and balance. These practices will help you to re-discover, strengthen, and find balance in your body, mind, and spirit.

In **Part Two,** I also share embodied voice explorations created by Arthur Lessac, famed originator of embodied voice, speech, and movement work called *kinesensics.*[5] This is where *The Postpartum Path of Yoga* is truly unique. *A program has never been developed for postnatal women that incorporates mindful healing and the development of the body, voice, and spirit.*

Think of embodied voice as "yoga for the voice" because you hone your awareness inward on your voice and speech. The Lessac work helps you develop vocal quality and clarity through a forward-focused, vibrant feeling voice so when you speak, you are clear, direct, and grounded in what you need to say. You can feel your voice as you speak because of the resonance of vocal vibration in the mouth. It grounds you. Whether speaking as an advocate, teacher, leader, or nurturer, you are authentic in expressing yourself. You have different qualities and dynamics in how you speak and relate to others because you have developed a range of expressive possibilities from the musicality of your speaking voice.

The way you discover the skillset of embodied voice becomes an emotional valve such that you can speak passionately about something and not lose yourself in heightened emotions at the moment. You will find new ways to make your point without needing to be loud and fatiguing yourself. "Embodied voice" means you have options for expressive dynamics that sustain your spirit and revitalize your body, mind, and voice again and again. The more you tend to it each day, this health and wellness practice will stay with you for life.

Each practice concludes with a meditation you can do whenever you have five minutes to sit and breathe—perfect for when you nurse or bottle-feed your baby! These meditations align breath, body, mind, and spirit; you return to your true self. Meditation leads you away from the small self that tends to suffocate you with the needs of the ego to the large self that is open-hearted, balanced, and connected with the Divine. Our practice together creates moments for mindfulness every time you breathe, move, and communicate, preventing "mommy burnout." *Moreover, the more you care for yourself, the better you care for your child.*

Remember, *The Postpartum Path of Yoga* focuses on more than physical well-being. It stresses the importance of building and fostering community with others experiencing similar life changes. I recommend using the seventh day of the week—the rest day—as a time to journal and work on the community-building idea posted at the beginning of each phase. Seek out women with whom to engage so you can heal your spirit.

Postpartum depression and anxiety are more common than mothers like to admit to one another. Even if they don't suffer from these conditions, the "baby blues" are real and speak to the painful isolation mothers feel when they abruptly stop the rhythm of their lives pre-baby by staying indoors and caring for a baby around the clock.

It's essential to find other wanderers similarly searching for connection, wellness, shared experiences, and a desire to integrate with body, mind, and spirit—individually and as a group. We need others to get through life's stressors, such as moving house or changing careers. Why should the experience of adjusting to the needs of a child and expanding our lives be any different?

Lastly, just as it takes time for meaningful friendships to form, it also takes time to deepen one's relationship with oneself. Mothers need to focus on self-care while acclimating to this new chapter in life. It's not a race; it's an endurance *adventure*.

PART THREE

Part Three leads you through a more advanced phase of the program once you have developed strength and stability in your core and hips. If you are a new mother, please complete **Part Two** at least twice before moving on to Part Three to ensure you have corrected many of the conditions I described in **Part One**. Even better, cycle through **Part Two** until your child reaches their first birthday to give yourself adequate time to let your body heal. If you are the mother of an older child upon starting *The Postpartum Path of Yoga* program, please complete **Part Two** at least once before moving on to **Part Three** to get to know yourself on a subtler level.

Part Three continues the program with three additional breath-based practices, stronger mindful movements that engage the core and hips, more advanced embodied voice explorations, and meditations. I begin each of the three weeks of **Part Three** with excerpts from the *Bhagavad Gita*, a sacred Indian text that teaches how to find your calling and honor Divinity within. Let these exceptions inspire your meditation practices and open your heart to self-inquiry and self-love.

PART FOUR

Part Four teaches the yogic truths for relating to yourself and the world. They're called the *yamas* and *niyamas*. You can let these writings be moments for deep inward reflection on how you relate to them as a woman and mother. Let them frame how you regard your daily practice. For instance, ask yourself if you are being kind to *yourself* in thought, word, and action as you move through a sequence. Are you being kind to others in how you think about them, speak to them, and relate with them?

You can complete **Part Four** simultaneously as **Part Two** or as a spiritual intensive once you have completed all six phases of the program. You will have completed your study of the *yamas* and *niyamas* before beginning **Part Three** if you are cycling through **Part Two** more than once to restore your body, voice, mind, and spirit. Take your time with the *yamas* and *niyamas*. These teachings can change your attitudes toward bodymind wellness and give you a handbook for how you create your life.

The Postpartum Path of Yoga brings a mother back to herself. The clarity you feel within radiates toward your child. You will feel vibrant and new. Similarly, you will feel dynamic and integrated with mind, body, voice, and spirit—the whole of YOU.

Reading this book begins a new season in your life. If you feel well, your child senses this energy and feels well, too. If you *know* your child feels well, you relax and find more joy in your daily life.

This cycle of wellness all begins with your embodied practice. Feel your breath. Get grounded. It all starts now.

~ 2 ~

PART ONE: THE FIVE CONDITIONS YOU DON'T HAVE TO ACCEPT

You may remember your third trimester of pregnancy: the shortness of breath from the fetus pressing on your heart and lungs, the lower back pain from the weight of your belly pulling you forward, and the instability in your pelvis, which may have led to waddling like a penguin. Perhaps your ob/gyn or midwife explained these happenings as you experienced them. Maybe you found ways to move and relax in prenatal yoga class. You may have read one of the many books on prenatal health and wellness and found them helpful.

Now that you've had the baby, you may find your lower back pain has bolted into upper back, neck, and shoulder pain. Your hips may feel unsteady, and you may have urinary incontinence when you jump or sneeze due to an imbalance in the pelvic floor muscles. You might feel loneliness unlike anything you've experienced before, which bewilders you. Unfortunately, no one may have explained the reasoning behind these occurrences. You may not have access to medical resources offered by your ob/gyn or midwife after the six-to-eight-week postnatal marker. Let the following be a light to lead you out of the darkness.

On Your Path Restoration

This section covers five physiological and anatomical conditions you can work through on your path to restoring your body, mind, and spirit. (Note: "Physiology" refers to the chemical livelihood of your body and mind; "anatomy" refers to the components making up your body.) My explanations of these conditions may help you better understand *how and why* you feel a particular way. Of course, all women are different and have various physical habits throughout their pregnancies. The state of your body postpartum depends on how you have lived through your pregnancy.

I'd like to offer information about these five conditions with a significant caveat: *You are not the summation of your parts.* You are a whole person with emotions, memories, passions, fears, intelligence, beauty, and love—to name a few of your qualities. The way you move encompasses all that lives *in* you and *as* you. Habitual ways of moving stem back to patterns and behaviors created unconsciously in childhood. With the practices in this book, you won't necessarily work to de-pattern these habits. Instead, you seek a relaxed yet curious, state of inquiry of body and mind. Then you can embrace and investigate yourself, noting discoveries as you navigate the work. Hopefully, you'll implement new ways of moving that encourage more healthful habits and behaviors, so you'll feel as well as possible.

That said, despite the beautiful complexities of individual women, physiological and anatomical givens are essential to understanding if we want to heal ourselves through intelligent movement-based practices. As trite as this saying may be, knowledge is power. Understanding the reasons for the physiological and anatomical changes in postpartum life brings about a sense of normalcy for how you may feel.

As you embark on a whole-bodymind program for restoring yourself, I'd like to share famed yoga teacher B.K.S. Iyengar's teachings on how yoga works to bring the practitioner to a spiritual connection. First, we come into a yoga pose (*asana*).

Our awareness is peripheral and on physical action at its most direct level...Next, we are doing the pose, all of a sudden the skin, eyes, ears, nose and tongue—all our organs of perception—*feel what is happening in the flesh*...The third stage...is when the mind observes the contact of [awareness on the periphery with what is happening within] and we arrive at mental action in the asana. The mind acts as a bridge between the muscular movement and the organs of perception, introduces the intellect and connects it to every part of the body...When the mind has come into play, a new thought arises in us. We see with attention and remember the feeling of action...We *discriminate with the mind*...[observing]...the feeling of the front, the back, the inside and the outside of the body...Finally, when there is a total feeling in the action without any fluctuations in the stretch...[all types of awareness and actions] meet together to form a total awareness from the self to the skin and from the skin to the self. This is the spiritual practice in yoga (emphasis added).[6]

Let this process illuminate your path as you learn about yourself, awaken parts of your body and voice that may have become dull from tension, revitalize these areas, and integrate your body, mind, voice, and spirit. You are working from the outside in and the inside out at once. Every new pose and exploration will bring you back to the periphery, and your work assimilates awareness with it and meets new information with what you know. Your powers of awareness, discernment, and concentration will grow stronger over time, aiding your meditation practice and enhancing your capacity to tune into your inner voice. Your physical and vocal practices may seem focused on rebuilding weakened parts of the body and voice, but they have more significant meanings for your spirit.

Remember that your body and mind function as a *complex*, which means one body part does not govern how the rest of the body and mind work. Instead, your whole self (body, mind, voice, breath, spirit) communicates and integrates as a beautifully intricate system. The more you feel this synergism, the more quickly you'll befriend and heal the bodymind. And the more you understand and connect with your physical body with a compassionate mind, the better you can care for yourself in other facets of your life, including how well you take care of your child.

The more you understand and connect with your physical body with a compassionate mind, the better you can care for yourself in other facets of your life, including how well you take care of your child.

Feeling better begets better self-care, which will positively influence your vocal and spiritual life. As you move through the program over time, you will move through your life with improved posture. This can further heal the parts of your body that were stressed by pregnancy and delivery. It all manifests into living your best life possible here and now.

Your Body as a System

Investigate how your body moves as a system. When you raise your arms overhead, you might feel a pull somewhere in the lower half of your body, like pulling a small section of a sweater and seeing a completely different part of the sweater move. It is impossible to move one part of the body and not feel sensation elsewhere if you are aware of the body's periphery. More interesting than that is how the body stores emotions, memories, and intellect. When you raise your arms overhead, you may have not only noticed a pull in the lower half of the body but also sensed a childhood memory of moving a certain way and felt an emotion tied to that memory or movement.

This happens because your nervous system communicates with your muscles when you feel muscles stabilizing joints and activating movement. Likely you move best when you feel good emotionally, which becomes an important piece of any wellness program: You must honor how you feel *emotionally* and *physically* sense movement. The more you move in a relaxed, steady, aware, and contented manner, the better your body (including your mind) will integrate what you discover about yourself.

CONDITION ONE: POSTNATAL DEPLETION TO POSTPARTUM
DEPRESSION AND ANXIETY

The first three months after a woman has birthed a baby are unlike any she'll experience. Commonly called the "fourth trimester," the infant adapts to the exterior world while the mother bonds with her baby and adjusts to her new role in life. Women change dramatically during this time. Even if your baby is not your first, you're now adapting as the mother of two (or more) children. Mothers wonder how they'll catch any meaningful sleep with a baby that wakes to eat throughout the night.

On the beautiful side, indeed, a woman's body is never the same once she bears and births a child. She now feels a love deep within that she never knew was possible. She finds ways to survive sleep deprivation for months because she loves her child so much and wants to comfort them through the night. Her physiology changes due to surges of oxytocin, the love hormone that gushes every time she and her child touch.

On the problematic side, the depletion of cortisol—the fight-flight-or-freeze stress hormone—rises with the difficulty of caring for her baby while feeling sleep deprived and anxious. In fact, around three o'clock in the afternoon, everyone commonly suffers a lowering of cortisol due to a fluctuation of the circadian rhythm. Most people reach for an afternoon sweet or caffeine boost to get through this dip in energy. Add to this the stress of putting the baby to sleep in the evening, when a mother's cortisol levels fall dramatically and leave her exhausted. Yet, the anxiety from the stress plus the afternoon caffeine/sugar boost prevents her mind from fully resting and bringing her to a restorative sleep. In addition, her upper back and shoulders ache from holding the baby for hours. She may feel isolated through the days and develop the "baby blues" or postpartum depression/anxiety, which worsens with a lack of sleep.

When they first care for their babies, many mothers suffer exhaustion, isolation, and depression with anxiety. These feelings can last for years. General Practitioner Dr. Oscar Serrallach calls this "postnatal depletion," which includes "feeling run down, lethargic, and battling often unexplainable chronic physical depletion."[7] This condition is physiological, emotional, and social.

Mothers face profound hormonal changes and feel social pressure to find the best mothering practices that align with societal expectations. They also lack the village of support mothers had a few generations ago. In addition, mothers are prone to postpartum depression if they assume they can handle a lot singlehandedly. It can also happen if their birth plan doesn't work out, as in my case. I wanted a vaginal birth but had to have a C-section.

Looking back, I am thankful for my C-section, despite how difficult my recovery was. Without it, I wouldn't have experienced the hardship that motivated me to learn more about myself, my anatomy, and my physiology. And I wouldn't have discovered the whole work that became this book. Thanks to my C-section, I have shared this work with women from all walks of life to help them heal. And let me mention my daughter, who entered this world via C-section and is the greatest joy I know!

Many postpartum depression sufferers feel ashamed because they failed to live up to their rigid expectations, which are based on an imagined societal standard. Moreover, sleep deprivation, stressed nutrition, and dehydration (especially if they are breastfeeding) are exacerbated, and mothers can spin into a downward spiral from there. Yet they do best when they are kind to themselves and are honest with what they can realistically manage.

Dr. Serrallach described postnatal depletion as a syndrome that arises as "the understandable outcome of a series of less-than-ideal events." He made these points:

1. The nutrients given over to making, incubating, and birthing the baby are enormous, and this depletion continues after the birth for breastfeeding women.
2. Bone-gnawing exhaustion can occur from sleep deprivation—the result of never having a good, refreshing night's sleep.
3. The drastic change of a new mother's role is often accompanied by social isolation, which can have a deleterious effect on a woman's psychological well-being.[8]

Postnatal depletion doesn't occur as a black-and-white illness but as a group of symptoms with varying shades of gray. How one mother feels six months postpartum may differ from how another feels at fourteen months postpartum, yet both may suffer from this condition. Moreover, the lack of self-care, sleep, and proper nutrition causes inflammation in the body, which leads to more inflammation the longer the mother continues to not care for herself. This is how postnatal depletion can last—sometimes, it takes years for mothers to find equilibrium again. (Don't worry; the program I offer in this book will help you start your path to self-care through the fog of postnatal depletion.)

Postnatal depletion can begin as soon as the placenta leaves the mother's body and last as long as a *decade*. McCulloch wrote:

> The placenta passes nearly 7 grams of fat a day to the growing baby at the end of the pregnancy term, while also tapping into the mother's 'iron, zinc, vitamin B12, vitamin B9, iodine, and selenium stores—along with omega 3 fats like DHA and specific amino acids from proteins ...' On average, a mother's brain shrinks 5 percent in the prenatal period, as it supports the growth of the baby (much of the brain is fat) and is re-engineered for parenthood.[9]

The placenta carries many nutrients for the baby, so its departure is an important physiological event. The placenta's absence in the body affects the pregnant woman's physiological balance because she used many of her body's nutrients to create it.

The brain shrinkage the mother endures once the placenta leaves could bring anxiety and postpartum depression. She may value taking care of the child's needs before considering her own. Yet, there may not be community support to help the new mother care for the baby and her home or make her meals.

Added to that, many mothers feel in competition with each other. Who had the most natural childbirth? Whose baby is breastfeeding the best? How long is the baby sleeping at night? Who is bouncing back more quickly than the other new moms? The questions run through contemporary society in the media and on the street. When you look at popular magazines, you'll see the stories of new celebrity mothers looking fit and enjoying life with ease and vigor, some as soon as four weeks postpartum. Who's to say there is any truth to these stories, but the message is loud and clear—mothers are somehow supposed to re-enter life with enthusiasm and vitality and with much of their baby weight gone. How can a new mother *not* put pressure on herself, either explicitly or subliminally, to do everything she can to meet these demands?

How can a new mother *not* put pressure on herself, either explicitly or subliminally, to do everything she can to meet these demands?

Mothers can deprive themselves of self-care and proper nutrition to give everything they have to their babies. Naturally, they want their little ones to thrive, so a new mother might refuse food, sleep, water, and trips to the bathroom to prioritize her child's needs. She can suffer extreme brain fog and have no help. Sleep deprivation brings about anxiety that hinders sleep, which causes worse brain fog and affects her nutritional choices. This continues in a downward spiral and demands an abrupt change in lifestyle to stop it, then work toward finding balance again.

Postnatal depletion doesn't only affect the mother but the baby as well. The rise of cortisol from lack of sleep, stressed nutrition, and postpartum anxiety overworks the sympathetic nervous system—the nervous system that carries a person through stressful events. So if the mother is stressed, anxious, or in a brain fog, she may not fully be able to tend to her baby's needs. In addition, cortisol can transfer through her breast milk to the baby, making the baby gain weight quickly and feel more nervous and less confident.[10]

Mothers need to know it's critical to lower their cortisol levels for herself and her baby's well-being. I recommend lifestyle changes to find balance again and stop the cycle of postnatal depletion. Relaxed breathing, meditation (even if for two-three minutes while steeping a cup of herbal tea or while nursing the baby), and time with a friend are wonderful practices for lowering cortisol levels. Laughing also lowers cortisol. And it can give a new perspective on an event, helping mothers find new reasons to chuckle at life's happenings!

Laughing helps mothers see an event through a new perspective and find a reason to chuckle at it!

Even better is to share a laugh with your baby when they discover something new and laugh at the joy of it. Once your cortisol levels normalize, you'll be able to sleep better, which will clear your mind and bring about better nutritional choices. Prioritize drinking water throughout the day, especially if you are breastfeeding. Sleep as much as you can when you are able. Sleeping and eating better will affect your digestion and capacity to enjoy an active life again. The triad of optimal nutrition, sleep, and activity will boost the benefits of each other and lift your spirit overall.

If you feel you suffer from postpartum depression and anxiety, some resources can help you. Please speak with your doctor about your concerns and explore appropriate routes for self-care, including medication if needed. If you feel you might harm yourself or your baby, please go to the hospital immediately for help. Postpartum depression and anxiety are legitimate illnesses that have a physiological basis. Please do not feel embarrassed or ashamed if you suffer from one or both conditions.

The Need for Community

The human need for relationships gets established as soon as a mother provides skin-on-skin contact, nutrients (mother's milk or formula), and shelter to her baby. This immediate satisfaction of survival requires established neurological programming for social connection to meet basic human needs. In his book *Social: Why Our Brains Are Wired to Connect,* Matthew D. Lieberman wrote:

> Food, water, and shelter are *not* the most basic needs for an infant. Instead, being socially connected and cared for is paramount. Without social support, infants will never survive to become adults who can provide for themselves. Being socially connected is a need with a capital *N* . . . Love and belonging might seem like a convenience we can live without, but our biology is built to thirst for connection because it is linked to our most basic survival needs.[11]

Satisfying our basic needs creates a foundational understanding of ourselves as worthy of care. This is self-actualization. Therefore, we can determine that a mother knows whom she is based on the quality of her relationships. If a child becomes securely attached to their caregiver, they have a framework of self-actualization as they relate to other people throughout life. Meaningful relationships matter in helping people understand who they are.

As you enter this new season of life as a mother, the relationships you sustain and those you develop strengthen your identity and sense of self. Shallow relationships with the grocery clerk or the coffee barista seen every other day don't do much to affirm your identity as a mother unless you happen to share stories about your mutual experiences. If you enter this new stage of life as a mother and have no relationships to connect about your baby and motherhood, how can you find your sense of self as a woman and a mother? Relationships come first; a personal sense of identity follows.

Relationships come first; a personal sense of identity follows.

Remember, as strong as we believe we are, we cannot develop our power and integrity independently. We need a community of people who understand us and our needs on some level. A group of new mothers provides the perfect network to find wellness support. Mommy/baby get-togethers could take the form of group yoga classes, La Leche League meetings, or mommy stroller walk groups. They can become important for a mother's physiological, emotional, and spiritual healing.

In every postnatal yoga class I have taught, I've worked with various women from different career paths, educational backgrounds, cultures, and religions. Despite the differences in the room, mothers come together with the commonality of being a new mother, not knowing what to do, and wanting to connect with other women. In every postnatal yoga class I teach, as the mothers share their ups and downs of motherhood, friendships form among them. If you don't have a yoga studio in your area with a trained postnatal yoga teacher offering such a class, do not worry. In **Part Two**, I provide community prompts to give ideas on finding a community of mothers and creating your tribe.

Dr. Amy Wenzel, psychologist, and expert in the field of perinatal distress, identifies three types of support—emotional, informational, and tangible:

> Emotional support is defined as the support experienced when a woman has a person or people who are truly there for her, providing her with warmth, care, and validation.

Informational support is defined as factual advice or resources that a woman can use in times of need. Tangible support is the actual help that a person can provide to a mother or family . . . A positive support system is the most critical part of a woman's recovery.[12]

Mothers can find emotional support in their partners, best friends, and family. If you don't feel close to family members, remember that we cannot choose the family we're born into, but we can choose who *becomes* our family. Best friends can fulfill that role and be ready to receive you when you need support.

You can also find resources online that offer help with questions regarding self-care or care for your baby. However, take online advice with caution and check the background of those who provide it. If you have medical concerns of any kind, please refer to your doctor/midwife or pediatrician for expert advice. Internet sources aren't valid for medical advice, nor are moms' groups on Facebook. Local friends, neighbors, and members of your place of worship can offer tangible support, so don't be afraid to ask for help. After my family had visited immediately postpartum, a woman from church brought a meal to my husband and me. Her home cooking felt amazing, and it was so lovely to feel cared for at that moment. An ounce of tenderness from someone can sustain your spirit a long way.

Her home cooking felt amazing, and it was so lovely to feel cared for at that moment. An ounce of tenderness from someone can sustain your spirit a long way.

You can also build a community network to expand your tangible and emotional support systems. If you take the time to search and follow up, you'll find many opportunities for mothers to meet and connect. It's better to seek in-person social time and connection rather than social media groups. Mothers often increase their anxiety via social media because of the inherent "mommy shaming" that occurs over one mother's choices for sleep training, bottle feeding vs. breastfeeding, and a dozen others that women make as mothers.

Remember, the point of being in a group is to make you feel better, not worse. If you feel anxious, sad, frustrated, or competitive in your social media group, leave it and seek out an in-person group. If there are no other options for interacting with mothers because you live in a remote area, post a handwritten sign on the local supermarket community bulletin board or library. State that you want to meet other new mothers in a shared public space for an hour of conversation. Start here and see where it grows.

CONDITION TWO: PELVIC FLOOR IMBALANCE

If you suffer low back pain, hip pain, constipation, or urinary incontinence, you may have an imbalance in the pelvic floor muscles. The pelvic floor cradles the organs of the lower torso and creates the base for deep-felt strength, balance, and stability. This area supports the load of pregnancy and then relaxes and stretches for the vaginal delivery of the baby. On an energetic level, the pelvic floor corresponds to the body's first energy center (called a *chakra*) and creates the foundation for our connection to our family. When the pelvic floor is out of balance, we feel unstable, weak, and disconnected from our essential needs. Once it comes back into balance, we notice how much stronger we feel and more convicted to do what's suitable for ourselves and our families.

Before diving into the particulars of the pelvic floor, first, let's understand how it relates and functions with the rest of the components of the core. With interest in understanding the anatomy of the postnatal body, let's start with the area that cradled and supported the fetus—the pelvis and the torso—and move onto the trunk of the body where its muscles connect at a particular point.

The pelvis comprises three main parts: the right side, the left side, and the sacrum. The top of the pelvis is called the "ilium." The bottom of the pelvis has two knobs commonly called the "sitting bones" or "sitz bones" for short. The bottom of the front of the pelvis is the "pubic bone," which has a ligament in the center, technically known as the "pubic symphysis." The back and center of the pelvis is a triangular bone/plate with ridges. It's called the "sacrum," which is part of the spine at the back of the pelvis before the spine ends at the "coccyx," also known as the tailbone. The location where the sacrum and the ilium meet on the right and left side is called the "sacroiliac joint," which contains ligaments and cartilage to allow for ease of movement in the pelvis and spine.

During pregnancy, the ligaments of the pelvis loosen due to the increase of the *relaxin* hormone, especially during the first trimester. This softening allows the pelvis to open and make room for the baby's descent through the birth canal. It also leads to pelvic instability and low back pain if there isn't sufficient core strength to support your body. Moreover, *relaxin* circulates through your whole body. It is safe to assume it affects more than the pelvis, but also impacts the wrists, shoulders, and other joint complexes. Moreover, *relaxin* stays in the body after you have had the baby for as long as you nurse your baby, and it can take up to four to five months to leave your system post-weaning. Although its effects on your body postnatally are not as predominant as when the baby is in utero, it's safer to assume gentler movement practices to preserve the integrity of the joints, particularly those in the pelvis, for five months post-weaning or five months postnatally if you are not nursing.

The "torso" is the area beneath the ribs extending down to the inside of the pelvic basin, including the front, back, and sides of the trunk. The abdominal organs live inside what's called the "abdominal sac." The abdominal sac is like a balloon; it has a natural amount of pressure inside, and its pressure can change based on how you stand, sit, breathe, and move.

The "thoracic diaphragm" is on top of the abdominal sac. Commonly known as the "breathing diaphragm," it is a muscle shaped like a mushroom cap and nestles inside the ribcage. The diaphragm *descends* involuntarily to fill your lungs with air and *ascends* as you exhale. We also have voluntary control over the diaphragm and can take a big breath to fill the lungs, thus, moving the diaphragm more deeply downward. The movement of the diaphragm directly changes the pressure of the abdominal sac, pushing it down and lengthening it upward as you breathe.

Focused breathing and moving in different directions during yoga class massage the organs in the abdominal sac. This becomes important to moving lymph and energy through your body as you work toward wellness. The diaphragm functions voluntarily and involuntarily. You can choose to inhale deeply, thus moving the diaphragm much lower than it would move on a relaxed breath. Whenever you breathe deeply, you give your organs an extra bit of massage downward and lift them when you exhale.

The pelvic floor is a diaphragm at the bottom of the abdominal sac. The muscles of the pelvic floor form a bowl shape and hold the internal organs of the pelvis and lower abdomen. Imbalances in the pelvic floor can lead to improper bladder function and con-stipation, among other complications. Specifically, the pelvic floor can become too tight or too slack due to poor posture, constricted breathing, or emotional tension. This can translate into muscular gripping of the pelvic floor openings-- the anus and the vagina. You may unconsciously tighten the pelvic floor due to a childhood memory, past injury, or childbirth trauma and not realize it until you work with awareness and breath control on releasing the pelvic floor. Poor pelvis posture comes from either tucking the tailbone or sticking the tailbone out, which compromises the integrity of the pelvic floor and tightens muscles, causing an imbalance. As you dis-cover postnatal wellness and balance through the practices in this book, work toward sustaining a neutral pelvis as much as possible (unless specified differently) while sitting, standing, and moving to equalize and balance the tone of the pelvic floor all around.

Work toward sustaining a neutral pelvis as much as possible while sitting, standing, and moving to equalize and balance the tone of the pelvic floor all around.

The pelvic floor diaphragm moves at the same time as the thoracic diaphragm. When you breathe naturally, and in a relaxed manner, both descend and ascend together. Due to this synchronized relationship, relaxed, yet focused breathing is an optimal way to treat a slack or tight pelvic floor. You can determine whether your pelvic floor is imbalanced by allowing your ob/gyn, midwife, or pelvic floor-trained physical therapist to assess you.

Once you have identified which way your pelvic floor is imbalanced (if you have an imbalance), then focus your awareness on either relaxing the muscles or toning them appropriately under the guidance of your pelvic floor physical therapist. A pelvic floor that is too tight needs a bit more focus on release and relaxation, while a pelvic floor that is too loose needs more contraction. Whether you have a pelvic floor that's too tight or too loose, pelvic floor contraction and release exercises (described in **Part Two**) will help bring *balanced elasticity* to these muscles. Over time, the pelvic floor will equalize, and you can spend the same energy and awareness on contracting and releasing.

Mothers might start a pre-pregnancy fitness regimen and notice those physical and physiological complications later: urinary incontinence when jogging or jumping, lower back pain, and extreme fatigue. *Caution:* Due to the higher probability of pelvic floor imbalance, the first six to seven months postpartum are not the time to start running or doing high-intensity interval training (known as HIIT) or begin other strenuous cardiovascular activities, especially while nursing. Please realize that your pelvis and surrounding muscles are still healing, and your hormone levels will take a while to regulate.

Also, if you do too much too soon after birthing a child, you risk raising your cortisol levels. This can hinder lactation, deplete your adrenal glands (causing fatigue), and inflame your muscles and blood vessels. Gentler yet comprehensive movement practices such as yoga and swimming are better choices than high-intensity exercises during your first six to seven months postpartum.

Gentler yet comprehensive movement practices such as yoga and swimming are better choices than high-intensity exercises during your first six to seven months postpartum.

Once your doctor or midwife has cleared you for exercise and yoga, they may recommend Kegel exercises to strengthen your pelvic floor. In a perfect world, the doctor or midwife will assess the condition of your pelvic floor and teach you how to properly perform them while also determining whether your muscles are too tight (hypertonic), too weak (hypotonic), or in balance. But I rarely see mothers in my yoga classes whose doctors or midwives have done this for them. Ask your caregiver to do this for you in your appointment, or at least ask how to perform the exercises they recommend for pelvic floor health properly. (If the doctor or midwife will not determine the pelvic floor's condition, seek a physical therapist specializing in pelvic floor rehabilitation. She can examine the pelvic floor, ascertain its state, and provide strengthening or releasing exercises along with the movements and practices in this book.)

Kegels are commonly understood as tightening and releasing the pelvic floor muscles. Although this is the inherent action of Kegels, many women need to consider the rhythm of the movement and how to perform the exercises with breath awareness. Doing Kegels isn't the wrong prescription; doing them incorrectly is.

People commonly describe doing a Kegel as stopping a stream of urine, holding it in, and releasing it. However, doing a contraction in this area is a tiny part of the practice to rehabilitate your pelvic floor and sustain optimal health. If someone recommends you practice pelvic floor contractions by stopping a urine stream, please know that this is not ideal. The pelvic floor needs to relax fully for the bladder to empty appropriately. Intermittently stopping the urine flow to engage in pelvic floor exercises can prevent your bladder from fully releasing the toxins the body has created. Over time, you can develop bladder infections due to bacteria lingering in the urinary tract. Instead, relax on the toilet and let nature run its course.

It is better to perform Kegels with mindful movement of the body synchronized with breath so your muscles move up and down freely. Because muscles are elastic, they perform best when they can contract and release with the breath and steady movement. Depending on whether your pelvic floor muscles are too tight or too loose, aim to balance these muscles with more focus on either the release or the contraction. Following a pelvic floor rehabilitation program is essential in postnatal life and beyond.

Depending on whether your pelvic floor muscles are too tight or too loose, aim to balance these muscles with more focus on *either* the release or the contraction.

Instead of calling this program "Kegels," I call it "Pelvic Floor Contraction and Release" (PFCR) to affirm the balance of energies of the pelvic floor. I suggest prioritizing your time investigating the pelvic floor, identifying the muscles, and noticing how they feel contracted and released. Then use this information for a daily practice of ten repetitions of long holds, then ten short pulses three times a day. You will fully relax the pelvic floor after each contraction. (More on this in **Part Two**.) The time you reserve for this initial inquiry establishes the awareness you need for your path onward.

Once you identify how to isolate the pelvic floor muscles to contract and release at will, create your training program. If you are short on time, you can double up duties by performing pelvic floor contractions and releases during stop lights while running errands. The couple of minutes you gain to practice each time you stop will add up nicely. You can also practice while nursing, feeding your baby a bottle, or snuggling with your little one. Remember that performing these exercises several times a day—even for one minute at a time—is *better* than negating them or doing them on the chance you remember. (We'll dive more deeply into identifying the pelvic floor and how to contract and release it appropriately in **Part Two**.)

CONDITION THREE: DIASTASIS RECTI

The most exterior layer of abdominal muscles is the "rectus abdominus," also known as the "six-pack abs," popularly built up from abdominal crunches. Diastasis recti is when the two vertical sheaths of the rectus abdominus separate unnaturally from the "linea alba," the band of connective tissue at the midline of the abdomen. Think of the plastic coin purses popular in the 1980s that were oval. They were opened by squeezing the two tall points of the oval toward each other, separating the midline, and allowing coins to go in or out of the purse.

For the rectus abdominus, the midline is the linea alba, and the purse is the abdominal sheath. Any slouching or spinal flexion puts pressure on both ends of the abdominal sheath, and the two halves separate. If left untreated, this separation could leave you unstable while moving your torso and cause back and/or pelvic pain. In extreme cases, over time, you can herniate through the separation from excessive intra-abdominal pressure brought on by misalignments from forceful movements (for example, sit-ups or lifting heavy objects).

Diastasis recti is a common condition not only for new mothers but anyone who endures misalignment of the ribs and pelvis in daily life. Some mothers are uncertain if they have diastasis recti because their doctors or midwives do not assess them during their six-to-eight-week postnatal checkup. However, you can determine this for yourself.

Start by lying on your back with your knees bent and feet on the floor. Relax and breathe naturally. Align your index and middle fingers and then place them just beneath the tip of the breastbone, pointing them downward toward the pelvis. *Slightly* curl the torso off the floor and feel if the *two* fingers descend into a gap. If they easily do, lie back down and place *three* fingers in the same place and repeat the curl-up. Repeat this using *four* fingers. This helps you determine the approximate distance of the separation. Depending on the number of fingers that descend, gently press them down the length of the abdomen while noticing the width of the gap. The gap will naturally be larger around the naval in this postpartum period. Ideally, it knits back together similarly to the linea alba of the upper and lower abdominal muscles as you heal. There will always be a small space between the two rectus abdominus muscles for the linea alba, so you can have functional expansion and compression of your abdomen.

Press your fingers down your abdomen from the tip of the breastbone to the pubic bone. Notice if the gap is wider at the upper abdomen or lower abdomen or if it's the same throughout. Relax the torso down, roll onto one side, and use your hands to help you sit up. You can repeat this assessment every eight weeks to determine how your rectus abdominus is healing. Ideally, there will not be a separation of more than one finger's width between the two abdominal sheaths. I recommend asking your doctor, midwife, or physical therapist who assesses your pelvic floor also to determine diastasis recti and offer recommendations for repairing it. (**Part Two** explores postural practices and gentle movements to help heal diastasis recti.)

CONDITION FOUR: A WEAK CORE

Many muscles surround the abdominal sac, but let's focus on the main muscles that compose what's commonly called "the core."

Muscles are elastic in nature—designed to expand and contract and move along the directions of the fibers that make them up.

Ideally, while moving in all directions and positions, we want to feel balanced and strong, yet flexible.

In the front and at the most recessive, or deepest, layer of the abdominal muscles and wrapping around the torso like a corset is the "transverse abdominis" or TA. This muscle attaches to the lumbar vertebrae at the lower back, wraps around the sides, attaches at the linea alba (the layer of connective tissue at the midline of the rectus abdominis muscle on the exterior of the abdomen), and attaches at the top of the pelvis and inguinal ligament. Furthermore, the TA connects with the breathing diaphragm beneath the lungs while the bottom of the TA attaches to the pubic bone.

The TA is called a "hugger" muscle because, when we exhale, it hugs *in* toward the deepest part of ourselves, thus assisting in exhalation. It braces to take on loads as we move, and it stabilizes the torso to prevent back and pelvic pain. This becomes important when we incorporate breathing practices into the movement practice for healing the abdominal muscles.

The "internal and external oblique" muscles are on the sides of the abdominal sac. The internal obliques lie between the TA and the external obliques. These muscles assist in breathing and moving the ribs and spine, with the external obliques also facilitating side bending. If they get too tight, the oblique muscles can pull on the most superficial layer of the abdominal muscles, the rectus abdominus. This will exacerbate diastasis recti (the split between the two halves of the rectus abdominus). Therefore, it is important to have as many opportunities to lengthen and release tensions in these muscles as it is to strengthen and tone them.

As part of any conditioning program, it's also important to lengthen the oblique muscles as well as strengthen them. This includes lengthening and releasing the muscles attaching to the hip on which you tend to carry your baby more than the other. You can find balance by lengthening it and breathing into it.

At the back of the abdominal sac lies the "multifidus," which is a muscle that runs through the neck, upper, mid, and lower back along the spinal column. These muscles stabilize the joint complexes along the spine and protect each vertebra. Poor posture tends to collapse the spine and, thus, weaken the muscles of the multifidus. Poor posture also leads to a collapse of the pelvis, which compromises the integrity of the pelvic floor. Do your best to stand and sit upright while evenly negotiating the weight of the items you carry (including your child) so you don't compromise your optimal posture.

Two other vital contributors to core health are the "iliopsoas" and the "adductors" muscles. The iliopsoas (pronounced "ill-io-soaz") muscles are made of two muscles: the "psoas" and the "ili-acus." The longitudinal iliopsoas muscles run on either side of the spinal column and attach to where the thigh bone meets the hip socket (the "lesser trochanter" of the femur).

The iliopsoas connects at the top with the central tendon of the thoracic diaphragm. This means constricted breathing can directly affect the health of the iliopsoas muscle. This muscle has several important functions, including flexing the hips and working as a weak adductor (thus, bringing the legs toward the body's midline). It's a critical walking muscle that can become weak with poor postural habits.

The adductor muscles are a collection of six muscles that run along the inside of the thigh and work to bring the leg back to the midline of the body. All six adductor muscles connect to the pubic bone in some way. Because the iliopsoas muscles and the adductors meet the pelvic floor at a certain point, they also contribute to pelvic floor health and stability.

Keeping the muscles in a healthy relationship with each other when you're in either a static or dynamic pose can inherently strengthen them. I say that because many people live with imbalance due to poor posture or misaligned movement patterns. That's why I encourage a mother to sit tall, finding length in her lower belly and lower back and rising from the breastbone upward through the crown of her head while also keeping the lower ribs engaged and down. These actions alone will lengthen your spine and increase the length of the four main groups that surround the abdominal sac's front, sides, and back, as well as the tone and balance of the pelvic floor. By feeling that the spine is long, you can stabilize and release your iliopsoas muscles due to the relationship between posture and breath.

By feeling that the spine is long, you can stabilize and release your iliopsoas muscles due to the relationship between posture and breath.

You can sit and breathe well whenever you nurse or bottle feed your baby, day or night. This means you can have a healthful practice anywhere, anytime, if you know the opportunities. A strong and stable core brings good posture, which facilitates optimal breathing. Better breathing helps regulate your cortisol levels (the fight-flight-freeze) hormone and reduce anxiety. You feel better about yourself because you feel more potent in presenting yourself to the world.

CONDITION FIVE: VOCAL FRY AND VOCAL FATIGUE

Have you ever noticed how your voice feels and sounds when you're exhausted? It feels low in energy and sounds gravelly. You might even feel or hear little pops or crackles when you speak, especially at the ends of sentences. This is called "vocal fry," a condition that happens when there is little breath support for vocalization and your vocal folds are kept in a tight position.

Let's look at our vocal anatomy to understand better what this means. In the throat are two vocal folds made of soft tissue. They vibrate when we speak and change their tautness based on our pitch (or how high or low we speak). We speak on an exhalation, but the voice doesn't get much support when our breathing muscles aren't optimally engaged or are simply weak. Once in the mouth, the voice vibrates against the bones in the skull for natural amplification. We encourage the vocal vibrations to move to placement near the front of the hard palate (or the roof of the mouth) by using the muscles in our lips and cheeks to encourage the voice to move to where it best resonates (or amplifies).

Assuming no pathological issues such as lesions or overworked vocal folds exist, vocal fry occurs when we speak with little vocal energy and minimal airflow. In these circumstances, we cannot feel vocal vibration moving forward in the mouth, which prevents the voice from resonating on the hard palate, teeth, and skull. As a result, the voice stays in the back of the mouth-- a more difficult place for vocal resonance-- we cannot feel the voice, and we can begin to feel disconnected from what we say.

Unfortunately, many people judge women who speak with vocal fry as unintelligent and emotionally imbalanced. Cate Madill, who directs the University of Sydney Voice Research Laboratory, researched the different perceptions of men and women who have vocal fry. She found that "women with croaky voices were perceived as more neurotic than men with croaky voices. Women with clear voices were perceived as being less neurotic as men with clear voices."[13] How can you avoid a croaky voice? You can come into your authentic self connected in mind, body, voice, and spirit by discovering your voice, finding its power and dynamic range, and expressing yourself through this extension of yourself. When working through vocal fry, speech and language pathologist Laura Purcell Verdun advises that "the focus is always on how to optimize or normalize vocal physiology for vocal production."[14] That means you want to feel your breath, work slowly and with loving kindness for yourself, and enjoy what you experience.

Feel your breath, work slowly and with loving kindness for yourself, and enjoy what you experience.

We develop a healthy range for the speaking voice by tuning into its sensations. Specifically, we feel vocal vibration in the bony surfaces of the hard palate, teeth, and skull. Others hear us through the vibrations and resonance we feel moving through air conduction. In this way, we help ensure people will hear us based on the richness and potency of the vocal vibrations we feel within the mouth. We feel more vibrant when we know others hear us clearly with a voice that is authentic and our own. We are not trapped in a voice that creaks and cracks, thus, weakening our spiritual connection to what we say.

As Arthur Lessac, famed voice and speech trainer and originator of Lessac Kinesensics, teaches, "You must avoid attempting to reach an audience, whether of one or thousands, by 'throwing' your voice. To do so creates tension in the body—particularly the jaw—that eventually results in vocal strain."[15] (**Part Two** features a range of practices that bring you to awareness of vocal vibration and strategies for developing natural vocal dynamics. These practices will simultaneously relax and energize you so you feel well inside and out when you speak.)

Through embodied voice practices, you will no longer feel strain in your throat when you speak to someone across the room. Happily, you won't feel weighed down energetically when you read a board book for the twentieth time to your baby (even when it's past your bedtime). That's because you will find ways to breathe and support your voice. You will enjoy the rhythms of language as you communicate with those around you. You will feel musicality in your voice and speech in ways that inherently feels nice to speak.

You will feel musicality in your voice and speech in ways that inherently feels nice to speak.

Developing vocal resonance strengthens the voice without straining the voice. It creates a potent, warm speaking voice that genuinely feels good. When I do a series of vocal resonance explorations, I feel like I have warm honey in my throat. It is completely relaxed, my voice is open and clear, and I speak effortlessly while feeling vocal vibrations on my upper gum ridge. When I feel my vocal vibrations on these bony surfaces, particularly the hard palate and upper gum ridge (where the hard palate meets the upper front teeth), I know people can hear me due to the amplifying nature of bones. If others can hear me, I don't need to shout to be heard. This honors a more peaceful balance of my energy.

Through this practice, I can emphasize an important lesson to my daughter and not scare her by shouting for emphasis. Instead, my vocal tone carries across the room. When communicating something urgent to her, its natural potency can match my dutiful, concerning body language, and she won't hear a shrill voice. As a result, she continues to feel safe and nurtured, which supports her self-esteem and personal growth.

Your Restoration Starts Now

Any of these five conditions could make you feel more detached from your essential self. They may exist independently of each other and may also feed into one another. B.K.S. Iyengar teaches, "The weakest part [of the body] is the source of action."[16] For example, your low back pain could result from a weak transverse abdominus and diastasis recti, which will compromise your posture, exacerbate your instability, and throw the rest of your body out of alignment as you move. This affects how you position your pelvis, further weakening the pelvic floor and destabilizing the core more, causing more low back discomfort. This could lead to difficulty sleeping, which worsens your fatigue during the day. This fatigue leads to poor breath support when speaking, which leads to vocal fatigue or vocal fry. Physical ailments can spiral downward energetically and worsen any symptoms of postpartum depression and anxiety.

So, here you are in this scenario, feeling isolated, physically in pain, and unstable when you move around. You also feel emotionally drained and have little impetus to express yourself with any dynamics that reflect your spiritual life. The low energy of those physical, mental, and emotional selves drags down your spiritual life, and everything perpetuates the cycle.

Instead, become aware of what feels weak as your inspiration for harnessing spiritual power when navigating your mindful movement practices. Now that you know where you feel unstable, you can focus here, spread your concentration peripherally through your body, and discover ways to share the load of the pose you explore. You can shift your awareness from one side of the body to the other. You can discern what feels great and what feels dull. The dull parts are weak, so you can put your awareness there. You can discover where you can engage your muscles or imagine breathing into these areas to awaken them. Your powers of concentration spread back to the bodymind as a whole, and you enter a state of meditation in the pose, which enhances your spirit.[17]

Despite the parts of you that feel compromised, there is hope. Please be aware of these conditions and how they affect you, then take the first step to improving only one. Feeling better will inspire you to heal the other conditions.

Please be aware of these conditions and how they affect you, then take the first step to improving only one. Feeling better will inspire you to heal the other conditions.

The moment you decide to make changes in your daily life to take care of yourself, you ignite a spiritual awakening in your deeply felt values that will sustain you from now on. It doesn't matter where you start—you just start.

The more you breathe optimally, the more you lower your heart rate. The more you lower your heart rate, the lower your cortisol levels become by pacifying the adrenal glands. The more your body feels peaceful, the more you can focus on your wellness and your child's well-being. When you attune with your child, you bond with them. You may feel a surge of love and warmth in these instances.

This is the effect of the oxytocin hormone—the love hormone—being activated from skin-on-skin contact and emotional attunement with another person.

If you ever feel anxious, stop what you're doing, breathe deeply, and feel where your body contacts the surface on which you stand, sit, or lie down. This is where you are grounded. Notice your heart rate lowering. If you are with your baby or child, hold hands and gaze into their eyes. Now soften your breath and gaze, allowing both of you to enjoy the benefits of oxytocin. The stronger the bond between mother and child, the more confident the child will develop over time. It all starts with your breath.

The stronger the bond between mother and child, the more confident the child will develop over time. It all starts with your breath.

Optimal breathing sustains your ability to remedy the five conditions that *do not* have to stay as you navigate being a mom to a baby. Moreover, the more mindful you become in your daily practice, the more mindful you will be of your sensations off the mat. This, in turn, will inform your decisions on how you eat and how much you move throughout the day. Your mindfulness for self-care will translate into increased and sustained energy and revitalized spiritual connections to those around you as you continue caring for your child.

Summary

These five conditions of body, mind, and voice may seem all-consuming, but they do not have to take over your life. You can rehabilitate yourself in body, mind, voice, and spirit. You will move beyond these conditions and come out stronger on the other side. Commit to yourself. Commit to the life you know is in store for you. Every ounce of focus and discipline you put into your restoration will grow exponentially for your future self.

~ 3 ~

PART TWO: THE PATH TO RESTORATION

Now that you know the five conditions you don't have to accept, let's step into what is readily available for you—vitality, expressive dynamics, and balance in body, mind, voice, and spirit.

Yoga is a wonderful modality that reaps many benefits. Many people feel intimidated by yoga because they see images of thin men and women in poses that require a lot of strength and flexibility. What they don't see is that many of those people may have hypermobile joints and may also nurse injuries sustained by doing the very poses they exhibit in the photographs! Yoga is *not* about putting your ankles behind your head, sitting with the tops of your feet crossed on top of the thighs, or sitting still for thirty minutes a day. It is *not* about comparing what you can do with what you see others doing. Here's what yoga is:

- a bodymind discipline that integrates awareness of physical sensations, movement of the breath, emotions, and state of mind (thoughts and temperament).
- a safe and appropriate means to nurture oneself in body, mind, and spirit because of how yoga balances and neutralizes the nervous system.

- a physical practice that stabilizes joint complexes over time, resulting in a stronger, more flexible, and more balanced body.
- a way to still the chatter of the mind such that one learns to observe the thoughts that come and go without getting lost or sidetracked into them. As a result, one becomes more responsive to stimuli and less reactive.
- a fabulous way to model self-care to children. When kids see Mama doing yoga, they can participate or watch. Either way, they see that Mama is important and worthy of care. Mama cannot take care of the family well unless she takes care of herself.
- accessible at any hour of the day in some capacity.
- a way of life that is honest, kind, value-driven, and vital with integrity and purpose.

Let's break these points down a bit. First, yoga is a discipline. It is something you tend to every day, whether it is for ten focused minutes or for an hour. The more you water this garden, the more you will see it grow. You will become accustomed to the practices you explore in this book, and they will become a way of life for you. As you explore yoga poses with kindness for yourself, you begin to treat yourself kindly when you are not practicing yoga. When you notice a racing mind in a yoga pose, you notice if you tend to have a racing mind in a situation in which you feel challenged. The more you seek balance in your mind as you explore a pose one step at a time, the better you will be able to follow a similar pattern in real-life situations. Moreover, optimal breathing practices become a way of breathing that keeps your emotions and thoughts balanced and connected to the moment every day.

Second, yoga is a safe and appropriate practice for everybody—and I mean every race, culture, gender, size, and type of body. If you can breathe, you can practice yoga. If you can move, you can practice yoga in some way (even if it is simply a meditation practice).

Yoga practitioners do best when they embrace where they are with kindness and move at a pace that keeps their joints safe. Bodies get stronger over time (and muscles need rest to rebuild, so pushing hard every day does you no good). Work in small increments, and you will see yourself getting more stable in poses with a fuller breath capacity than you had last week. You need to commit to the process and show up for yourself to see it through. Working with equanimity helps to balance the nervous system because your slower, more measured breathing practice calms cortisol levels in the body, reduces inflammation, calms the mind, and stimulates the vagus nerve, thus promoting a healthy parasympathetic nervous system (which brings us a state of peace and safety from within).[18] The body can balance hormonal levels in a more restorative framework free from inflammation.

Third, yoga stabilizes joint complexes over time because you build strength by holding poses for five full breaths (inhale and exhale). The key here is to resist collapsing into a pose; instead, lengthen through it, feel the shape of your body from the inside out. Stay connected from your feet through the crown of your head, and you will notice muscles activating to support your posture and alignment. This activation stabilizes joints and strengthens the muscles that surround them.

Fourth, yoga quiets the mind to one of focused thought observation. Meditation is a key component of yoga practice, even as you move from pose to pose. Finding a single point of focus outside of you [called a *dristi* (pronounced "drish-tee")] helps you withdraw your senses towards the point you see and the sound and feel of your breath. If you explore a seated meditation practice, you find a soft gaze with your eyes or close your eyes and feel your breath moving in and out of your body. You might focus on a word or short phrase (called a *mantra*). Other thoughts will come. This is natural and to be expected. The discipline is in observing those thoughts without getting lost in them. For example, if you sit in meditation and focus on your breath, you may get thoughts about the grocery shopping you need to do, the laundry waiting for you in the dryer that needs folding, and the supplies you need to pick up from the craft store for your child's science project. You are human, a mother—of course, you have a list of things to do! However, can you observe the thoughts and say, "Thank you, I will tend to you later," and imagine brushing them to the side and tending more fully to the breath itself? You will not forget your list, do not worry. Instead, you will develop a way to honor the tasks in your daily life while also keeping self-awareness at the center of your mind. In this way, as you complete the tasks in your life, you will develop an awareness of how you feel as you execute them such that you are still observing the thoughts that come and not reacting to them immediately. This does not mean you become robotic. Instead, you become more vital and human because you are present and connected with yourself in your surroundings!

Fifth, yoga is a great way to model self-care to your children. If you have a baby, lay the baby down for tummy time or on their back next to you and let them watch you practice. Give a loving gaze as you are able. Give a kiss when you can. But get back to your practice and let them see you take care of yourself. If your child is older and they interrupt your practice, calmly say, "Mama's doing yoga right now to take care of herself. I can help you in a few minutes." Complete the pose safely, conclude the meditation or the embodied voice practice, and know that you can return to it at your next opportunity. By not jumping up instantly to help your child (unless there is a true emergency!), they learn that Mama is important, too, and will be more available to help because she has helped herself. I cannot stress this enough: *you must model how to take care of yourself for your children.* They will need these skills for self-regulation and self-care as they become adults. Let them see how it is done, and they will know you are sincere when you suggest these tools to them the next time they are upset.

Sixth, yoga can happen at any time. You can practice optimal breathing at red traffic lights. You can meditate while you wait for the morning coffee to brew. You can explore a movement practice and an embodied voice practice while your child naps or is at school for twenty minutes or longer. You can meditate as you lay in bed before going to sleep. You can hum your consonants as you speak to keep a bodymind connection to your voice. Truly, the possibilities are endless. Once you embrace this, you will not feel time-constrained to practice yoga! The only limitations are the ones in your heart and mind. Please release them and see what life is like when you sprinkle a yoga practice throughout the day as you are able.

Last, yoga is a way of life rooted and framed by ethical living. These ethics are kindness, honesty, only what you need, releasing excess, conserving your energy for what matters, cleanliness, contentment, adopting practices that challenge stale habits holding you back, self-study, and surrendering to the flow of life. There is only so much one can plan—it is much better to experience life as it comes within the framework of your life with your family. Enjoy it moment to moment, and let yourself be surprised by your adaptability, sense of humor, and inner strength.

Tenets of a Yoga Practice

Yoga practice is more than breath, poses, and meditation. An ancient yoga sage named Patañjali transcribed an eight-limbed path to yoga, or union with body and mind, in the *Yoga Sutras*. The eight limbs are:

1. the *yamas*, or ethical guidelines to relating with the world
2. the *niyamas*, or the ethical guidelines for taking care of yourself
3. *asana*, or the postures and poses of the movement-based practice
4. *pranayama*, or breathing practices, including breath control and retention

5. *pratyahara*, or withdrawal of the senses so we are not distracted by the outer world but more readily able to tune inward

6. *dharana*, or concentration on our breath, inner sensation, and/or movement

7. *dhyana*, or meditation

8. *samadhi*, or complete integration of body, mind, and spirit.

In our movement-based practice, we practice each of these limbs on the yoga mat. Notice your thoughts as you practice yoga asana—Are you critical of yourself? Are you pushing yourself too far into poses and compromising your safety? Are you impatient with yourself? Once you recognize how you regard yourself, you can correct these thoughts with ones that support and nurture you.

Rick Hanson writes in *Buddha's Brain* how our brains are wired for survival by recording bad situations, pain, and disdain so we can learn about danger and work to avoid it. This served us thousands of years ago when we directly shared the land with beasts. Today, we record trauma and hardship from our life experiences and are quick to judge ourselves and others to avoid embarrassment, conflict, and strife. Hanson writes how this "negativity bias...generates an unpleasant background of anxiety, which for some people can be quite intense...The negativity bias fosters or intensifies other unpleasant emotions...highlights past losses and failures and downplays present abilities, and exaggerates future obstacles."[19] We can choose to rewire the neural pathways of the brain, so we do not automatically resort to an anxious thought that launches us into an unpleasant experience. Hanson proposes several strategies. One is to foster positive experiences in the moment of an adverse happening. For example, imagine you are in a yoga pose and feel embarrassed because you cannot do the pose like the teacher demonstrates, eliciting shame from childhood trauma or fear. At this moment, you feel your body grow heavy and clumsy, and emotionally awkward.

In this very instance, actively search for something—anything—positive that is also happening. Your feet feel grounded, you are proud of yourself for coming to the class, or you enjoy the feel of your outfit. Dive into the positive experience. Next, savor the experience for at least five seconds. The longer you stay with it, the better you will re-write the neural pathways in your brain. Hanson teaches, "Focus on your emotions and body sensations since these are the essence of implicit memory. Let the experience fill your body and be as intense as possible."[20] Relax your body and absorb the positive experience. You have now worked towards re-wiring your brain's neural pathways and creating new thought patterns.

If you meet a tricky pose, you may not immediately feel ashamed that you cannot do it. Instead, you may focus on how good your feet feel as you ground your awareness through them or how your body feels exploring the pose. You may feel curious and compassionate for yourself because you carried positivity from your previous experience to this moment. These neural pathways inform how you relate to life off the yoga mat: instead of feeling embarrassed or ashamed for not knowing how to do something, you may find yourself balanced and receptive to learning.

Hanson's recommended practice helps us discern when we strive too much and resist the natural flow of the moment. Notice how you breathe in your yoga practice—are you breathing heavily? This is an indication that you are pushing too hard. How can you ease out of the effort and find a nice balance of work and relaxation in the poses? Similarly, how can you find this balance in your daily activities? Do you tend to overwhelm yourself with tasks on top of the already tiring job of motherhood? Sometimes we do not have a choice—we have to work careers while also nurturing a family. However, when can we layer in moments to breathe optimally? You can easily layer in five breath-centering practices in your day—when you rise, before each of your three meals, and at bedtime. Even better—breathe optimally at every red traffic light and when you need to use the bathroom. These moments of mindful breathing can reset your nervous system and sustain your energy throughout the day to prevent burnout.

The more we center our awareness on how our breath feels within, the easier we can withdraw the senses time and again to balance the nervous system. Notice how jarring it is to scroll through social media on your phone, read the news on your computer, listen to the radio, and eat overly processed foods laden with sugar, salt, and fat. It is genuinely sensory overload. Lighten your sensorial intake by eating as many whole foods as possible, resisting the urge to check your phone for text messages or social media notifications (this is truly an addiction worth tending to in your meditation practice), and work to read or hear about the news once a day. Choose to keep an inward focus as you navigate the day so you can monitor how you feel as you relate with the world. If you feel burnout coming on, take a moment to close your eyes, breathe, and connect with yourself.

Meditation in small pockets of time turns into a larger capacity for concentration. You will find you are better equipped to focus on projects and be present with your family. More importantly, meditation hones your capacity to hear and respond to your inner voice. Sitting comfortably with your eyes closed places you at the center of yourself, regardless of what state you are currently in. Sit, breathe, and get to the heart of what is going on with you. You will find stillness at the base of every inhalation and exhalation—this is your spirit. Connect with it and ask it a question now and again that can help clarify a larger intention for your life. You will begin to hear your inner voice share with you what you need to do to do your best work in this life. I am not talking about work as your career. Instead, this work is why you are on this beautiful Earth. You can find your calling and your purpose through meditation practice. In yoga, this is called your *dharma*. Once you feel it, you feel amazing the more you pursue it. Listen to your inner voice, note the actions you need to take to serve yourself and others in your highest good, and get into spiritual alignment with your thoughts, words, and actions. You will feel free and light as you explore your true path.

Lastly, we feel *samadhi*, or complete integration, in daily life when we are less reactive to the world and more connected and relating with the world. You will react negatively less and less when your child raises their voice at you in a plea for help or to assert their independence. You will feel you live a life of integrity when you know in your soul that you are honest with how you care for yourself in healthful ways that, in turn, also support your family's health. You will feel more adaptable/flexible in your family's plans and will more and more bear witness to whom your children become as they grow into adults instead of pushing them into a design of your creation. This will also teach them how to stand in their light and find their path because you have modeled it for them through your daily yoga practice as a lifestyle.

Beginning a Yoga Practice in the First Year Postpartum

Having a baby is undoubtedly one of the most remarkable events of a woman's life. You experienced the miracle of pregnancy and your body's wisdom to develop and grow a human being inside of yourself. You delivered your baby and suffered pain like no other, regardless of whether your baby entered the world by vaginal or Caesarean birth. You held your baby for the first time and officially launched the rest of your life in a completely new identity: Mama.

The first fourteen weeks postpartum are considered the "fourth trimester." It is when your baby adjusts to being in the outside world, and you feel your stride as a mother. You will be exhausted, physically depleted, dehydrated, and experiencing mixed emotions daily—sometimes several at once! You should rest as much as possible during the first six-to-eight weeks of the fourth trimester. Focus your energy on your nutrition, breathing well and in a relaxed manner, walking when you can, and enjoying as much skin-on-skin contact with your baby as possible. If breastfeeding, this is a wonderful time to massage the area around the breasts to relax the muscles around the chest and shoulders to help facilitate lactation more easily. If you had a C-Section, begin massaging your incision site six to eight weeks after surgery to break up scar tissue and befriend this area of your body. The texture you feel will not be as smooth as an area that hasn't been surgically cut, but don't let that disturb you. Work gently. Breathe through the massage. Once you can explore the *Movement-Based Practices*, be kind to yourself if you feel pulling on that region of your abdomen. In this instance, lessen your range of motion, breathe deeply yet naturally, and slowly work toward lengthening the muscles and fascia in the area that feels the pulling through your postural alignment. Over time, you will be able to increase your range of motion again and build mobility in that area.

You are cleared for a yoga movement practice once your ob/gyn or midwife determines you are fit to do so. You may feel anxious to start flowing through Sun Salutations if you experienced yoga pre-pregnancy, but it is important to ease into your practice. Your body is very different than what it was pre-pregnancy and during pregnancy. If breastfeeding, you still have the *relaxin* hormone circulating through your body, which increases your joints' flexibility. You do not want to overstretch your joints and ligaments by doing too much too soon.

In my postnatal yoga classes, I focus on meditation, connecting with the baby through baby massage and gazing, and stabilizing the core, pelvic floor, and muscles around the pelvis so the ligaments can heal appropriately. This means I keep the left and right sides of the pelvis balanced as much as possible throughout the class, and we focus on strengthening the hips and legs with many of the explorations I list throughout this program. I do not include lunges or standing Warrior poses at this time because they move the two sides of the pelvis in opposition to each other. Besides, women already experience this movement when they walk, which is fine, normal, and great for the pelvic floor. I do not see any need to exaggerate this movement of the pelvis in a yoga class with longer holds. I'd instead focus our time on stabilizing the pelvis.

Similarly, I do not do kneeling or full planks in the first year since most women experience some degree of diastasis recti in the first year. If there is an abdominal separation, the intraabdominal pressure built up in planks can aggravate the mid-to-low back and encourage urogenital herniation. Likewise, any abdominal curl-ups risk the same effect on the body. You may also see "coning" in these postures, which looks like a concentrated bulge in a pyramid shape coming out of the midline of your abdomen while you're in a kneeling plank or lying on your back with your spine slightly flexed or rounded. Don't worry; having belly fat hanging down due to gravity is natural and nothing to fret about. There are safer ways to strengthen the core muscles, and I teach explorations that stabilize and lengthen the muscles surrounding the core's cylindrical shape so you feel balanced and strong overall.

It's best to do movements (listed below) geared toward toning the transverse abdominus with a gentle contraction of the pelvic floor muscles for core stability. These explorations include *Table Pose* with awareness of the length of the spine and breath awareness of the fullness of the exhalation, *Bird Dog Pose* with a similar awareness to *Table Pose*, and any poses in which I cue the length of the spine and alignment of the body regarding balancing awareness to all sides of your core.

You will find we focus a bit more on the physical body in the first few months postpartum as you embark on this program. Although we honor the eight-limbed path and recognize movements for the physical body are only one of them, it is hard even to recognize your spirit if you are in pain, exhausted, or suffering a myriad of aches caused by any of the five conditions explained in **Part One**. These physical distractions make it hard to investigate how energy moves within or how you feel when you meditate on any meaningful level. As a result, we concentrate on restoring the physical body as a temple for the spirit that resides within. Let's repair, renew, and rebuild the body, so we feel balanced and well to dive more deeply inward.

Breathe well, move intelligently, feel and develop your voice as a woman and mother, and explore a meditation practice to enhance your daily life. You will cultivate inner and outer strength supporting stronger practices in the second year of postpartum life.

The Importance of Yoga Props

We use yoga props for the *Movement-Based Practices,* so you get the support you need to build strength safely. I recommend investing in these yoga props to help you find optimal alignment in the poses: a sticky yoga mat, one or two firm folded blankets (wool blankets are best), two yoga blocks, and a six-to-eight-foot yoga strap. You can find yoga mats at most discount retail stores. I recommend thicker mats for joint comfort. You can find good quality mats online that will last over a decade. You can easily find blocks and straps at discount retail stores, and you'll find yoga blankets from online retailers. If you suffer knee pain or strain in any seated pose with your knee bent, place a block between the bent knee and the floor to prop it up. For standing forward folds, yoga blocks are wonderful. They raise a flat surface for you to ground your hands onto. Yoga straps are also helpful extensions of your arms for any pose in which the idea is to hold the opposite hand behind the back (for example, *Cow Face Pose*).

Most importantly, if you need to opt out of practice to take care of your child, yoga props can become an essential tool for nursing/ bottle feeding your baby while you attend to your breath with safe, mindful movement. Always sit on a folded blanket for optimal alignment between your shoulders, rib cage, and pelvis. Alignment means your shoulders are relaxed and down, your rib cage is evenly aligned above the pelvis with the lower ribs engaged toward the spine so your upper belly and mid-back feel equal length to each other, and your pelvis is evenly grounded on the blanket. Your lower back is lengthened, not slumped, with your pelvis tucked underneath you. Use blocks under your arms to support your baby by placing them between your thighs and forearms. Also, lay a folded blanket on the blocks for extra height and padding. Yoga bolsters make wonderful props for supporting your baby while you feed them if you can add one more prop to your collection. They become a fabulous investment you can often use, either while feeding your child or for your at-home yoga and meditation practice.

Guidelines for Your Path

My focus for the first year postpartum is to practice kindness for yourself, and learn about yourself in this new phase of life. Even if this baby is your second, third, or fourth, you are a new mom to *this* baby and are discovering how you relate to this circumstance in your life. I highly recommend finding a friend to practice with. Did you meet another pregnant mama from your ob/gyn or midwifery practice? Even if her due date differed, invite her to practice with you. Make a friend at story time at the public library and invite her over. If you are a mother of an older child, invite other mothers you know to practice with you while your children play. Building community is important to your restoration of body, mind, voice, and spirit.

Your path moves through six phases: The first two each last two weeks and the next four each last three weeks. You may find similarities between what you completed during one phase and what you will embark on next. This is to ensure your bodymind learns how to move safely, breathe, and sustainably.

Each week of the phases is launched with yogic teaching. Think of each of these teachings as a touchstone for your practice week after week. Spend time with them and see how they resonate with you. Experiment with various times of day to explore your practices.

I recommend completing the *Breath-Based, Movement-Based,* and *Embodied Voice Practices* all at one time as an integrated program.

It's lovely to complete your daily practice with meditation, but if you are pressed for time, you can meditate before you go to bed—making sure you stay awake!

Meditation works best when your mind is relaxed yet engaged with your inner sensations. If it's too difficult to meditate in the evening, do it during your baby's first nap or while your older child is at school. The more you commit to the discipline of personal growth, the more naturally time will become available for you.

The more you commit to the discipline of personal growth, the more naturally time will become available for you.

Let's explore three grounding guidelines for your practice:

First, throughout the practice and daily life, find relaxed and natural breathing as much as possible (unless the *Breath-Centered Practice* directs you otherwise). The more you breathe into a relaxed abdomen, the more relaxed yet focused your mind will be. For the first six to seven months postpartum, focus on meditation, natural and optimal breathing, and optimal alignment of your spine with your pelvis. This will help lower the cortisol levels in your body and increase the oxytocin levels that keep you feeling safe, thus ensuring your child's safety. Natural and optimal breathing and lowering of cortisol levels also facilitate lactation for breastfeeding mothers.

Second, when you are doing the *Movement-Based Practice*, work to keep moving steadily as you shift between poses. Do not bounce or jump from pose to pose as you may have done in pre-pregnancy yoga classes (typically vinyasa flow classes), because it could destabilize the pelvic floor upon impact. Please consult your doctor or midwife before beginning any movement-based daily practice.

Many mothers seek a good stretch to work out binding kinks in their yoga poses. But I'd like to change the way of thinking about "stretch." First, a stretch has a limit before it breaks. For example, if you stretch a rubber band far enough, it's bound to snap. Thus, using the word "stretch" regarding your body is not the kindest image. What if you instead think of *expanding* the muscle you seek to open? The idea of expansion invites you to breathe as you move, facilitating the openness you seek.

Better yet, I encourage you to think of *releasing* while you move. Breathe into your tight shoulders and then release your breath into the area that needs a bit of love. Feel your breath expand your chest and release your shoulders as you breathe. Feel the tension dissolve. *Release* the "story" you put onto your shoulders (e.g., "My shoulders are so tight because I had to carry two loads of laundry up and down the stairs without any help."). Release the breath, the tension, the story. Just let them go and focus on *what feels good* as you breathe, move, and connect with yourself and your child.

Release the breath, the tension, the story. Just let them go and focus on *what feels good* as you breathe, move, and connect with yourself and your child.

Third, I advise the breast-feeding mothers and those bottle-feeding less than five months postpartum to honor the pelvis's healing by limiting the length of your stride to 50-70% of what you'd *initially want to do* regardless of sitting or standing. Be conservative! Do any poses that open the hips (*Seated Wide-Legged Pose, Cobblers Pose, Goddess Pose*) at 50-70% of your range of motion and, to discourage hypermobility, shorten the stride between your legs. Be sure to focus your yoga practice on relaxing, strengthening, and safely conditioning all the core, including the pelvic floor.

Be sure to focus your yoga practice on relaxing, strengthening, and safely conditioning all the core, including the pelvic floor.

An Explanation of the Embodied Voice Practices
The *Embodied Voice* explorations over the six phases will produce vocal clarity, a warm feeling to the voice, and vocal health overall.

Strive for vocal clarity by feeling the musicality of consonants as you explore their tactile nature in your mouth as you speak. Vocal resonance—the richness of the voice as it vibrates in the bony surfaces of the mouth—includes the vibration of the voice in the skull that becomes a natural amplification system. Vocal tone will more easily waft forward to these bony surfaces if we feel a slight forward-moving action of the lips and cheeks in addition to a slight yawn-like action of the back of the throat (as if you are about to yawn).

Arthur Lessac calls this action the "reverse megaphone"—it's like a megaphone that begins at the lips and extends outward but in reverse.[21] The opening of the megaphone is at the back of the throat, the cheeks, tongue, and hard palate make up the sides, and the lips are *slightly* forward as if gently shushing your baby to sleep.

Explore the opportunities for vocal resonance within the space of the reverse megaphone and notice how much fuller your voice feels and sounds. But rely more on the *feeling* of your voice than the outer ear, which is not a reliable tool for independent voice training.

Rely more on the *feeling* of your voice than the outer ear, which is not a reliable tool for independent voice training.

Work to explore your voice with dynamic behavior so the explorations do not become mechanical. Be curious about your voice. If you need to, do the work as if vocalizing to your child with a twinkle in your eye. You risk regarding yourself as a body with parts and not as a whole expressive being if the work becomes mechanical. Putting behavior in your explorations while working mindfully frees the breath, attracts your interest, is fun, and develops your voice all at once. If you're working toward heightening your sense of self, you need to engage with what you're doing, so you can continually manifest wellness for yourself every time you move and speak.

In **Part Four**, you will have the option of navigating the ethical guidelines for connecting with others and taking care of yourself (called the *yamas* and *niyamas)* concurrently with **Part Two**. Doing so may deepen your understanding of these guidelines for living, and you can apply these lessons to how you move through the practices in each phase. This is optional—you can focus on **Part Two** and move through **Part Four** once you've completed **Phase Six**.

Yoga becomes your life in the most magnificent and liberating way possible. Yoga is a daily practice of inner strength and conviction to your values (which you discover in meditation) and flexibility in supporting yourself and your family. Life is a fluctuation of happenings, and the more we can ride its waves with equanimity, the better equipped we are to navigate storms and enjoy the peaceful times in which we can bask in the beauty surrounding us.

Our opening *yoga sutra* for **Part Two** is *Athayoganusasanam,* which translates as "Now we begin the study of yoga" (*Yoga Sutra* 1.1). It's a declaration of starting. Find your focus, feel your breath, and let's begin.

Phase One

For most people, (deep insight into complete absorption of the heart-mind) is preceded by faith, vitality, strong memory, samadhi, then deep insight.
Yoga Sutra 1.20

Start by finding faith at the beginning of your path. Trust that you will be creating something that serves the greater good—your wellness, your baby's wellness, and spiritual integration with body, mind, and voice that lifts you throughout all the days of your life.

Over the next two weeks, we will create the foundation for identifying sensation, understanding the pelvic floor, experiencing the synergy of breath and movement, and establishing healthy postures that support your movements and breath on and off the yoga mat. Your breath-based practice and meditation will hone your awareness inward. That way, you can quiet the mind, better feel sensations, and discover your inner landscape. Your embodied voice practice will connect you with the natural musicality of voice and speech.

Community Prompt

Reach out to a friend and see if they can stop by for a visit. Make a cup of herbal tea and enjoy each other's company while they meet the baby and chat about how you are doing. Allow yourself to be honest with your friend and yourself in your discussions.

Phase One, Week One

Breath-Based Practice: Finding Awareness with Breath

Lie with your knees bent and your feet hip distance from each other. Let the knees fall toward each other in a position called "constructive rest." You want your body to be relaxed so your mind can soften.

Tune your awareness inward to your breath. Feel it coming in and out through your nose. Notice its temperature and where you feel your breath moving your body, particularly your chest, belly, sides, and back. Notice this movement without judging it. Just be one with it and enjoy the sensations of breathing.

Now imagine you are smelling something you genuinely enjoy. Breathe it in with pleasure. Exhale a sigh with the satisfaction of having smelled this wonderful aroma. Arthur Lessac calls this exchange "pleasure smelling" and "pleasure sighing" to elicit wonderful relaxation in the body and mind while you explore the breath. Continue *pleasure smelling* and *pleasure sighing* as you attune with your breath. After ten cycles, return to natural breathing.

Movement-Based Practice: Foundational Practices

Become aware of upright posture and breath for these two seated practices whenever you can sit on the floor to relax and be with your baby: *Staff Pose* and *Easy Pose*.

Staff Pose, *Dandasana*

- Sit on the edge of a firm, folded blanket and extend your legs straight ahead. You can space your ankles a couple of inches apart from each other.
- Flex your feet like you are standing on them and feel as if you are floating through the crown of the head.

- Press your hands down on the blanket on either side of your hips. Feel that the lower belly is as long as the lower back and engage the deep core muscles from the pubic bone up to stay active in the pose.
- Breathe five breaths.

Whenever you want to reestablish your pelvis/ribs/head postural alignment, *Staff Pose* is a good neutralizing pose to return to throughout your practice. Explore *Easy Pose*.

Easy Pose, *Sukhasana*

- Sit on the edge of one or two folded blankets to prop up the sitting bones at the base of the pelvis. Feel the lower back lengthen with the length of the lower belly.
- Comfortably cross your shins and feel your spine lengthen. Keep your belly soft and breathe naturally.

Notice the difference between *Staff Pose* and *Easy Pose*. You want to feel the same core engagement and upright posture with a sense of rooting down through the base of the pelvis and floating up through the crown of the head as you did in *Staff Pose*. If you feel a collapse in your core, sit on another folded blanket and place a yoga block under your knees or thighs to support them. Breathe easily here, then explore ten pelvic floor contractions and release exercises (ten long holds, then ten short holds).

A note about Easy Pose: Notice which shin typically lays in front of the other while seated in this pose. Then consciously change the cross of your legs every time you sit this way. Sitting in this pose with your legs in the same cross will delay the ligaments of your pelvis stabilizing to where you can safely regain strength in your hips over time. If you normally sit with your right leg leading, next time, change to sitting with your left leg leading for the same number of minutes. Then the next time you sit in this pose, go back to the right leg leading and switch to the left leg leading the following time, and so on.

If you feel imbalanced with the other leg leading, sit on the edge of one or two thick folded blankets so your knees are at the same height as the ilium (top of the pelvis). If your knees are almost on the floor in this pose, try sitting with yoga blocks or a rolled towel under your thighs to prop up the legs so your knees line up with the top of the pelvis. This way, the ligaments can work toward healing without being pulled downward by the knees.

If *Easy Pose* does not feel comfortable because of a strain in your hips, low back, and/or knees, come out of it. Then kneel on a folded blanket between your calves and sit on it as if it were a bolster. If your blanket isn't thick enough to support you comfortably, then place a yoga block on the lowest setting with its width between your calves. Know that the base of your pelvis is about as wide as the width of the yoga block. If this feels better for you, kneeling is a better practice than *Easy Pose*.

The following exercises make up what I call the *Core Foundation*:

Pelvic Floor Contraction and Release—Identifying the Pelvic Floor

Now that you have connected with the flow of your breath, let's carry this over to identifying the pelvic floor and how it contracts and releases with the movement of your breath. You may remember from **Part One** that the pelvic floor diaphragm moves in sync with the thoracic diaphragm. As you breathe in, both diaphragms descend; as you breathe out, both rise. It's important to understand where the pelvic floor is, how to contract it correctly, relax it, and help it regain elasticity properly.

- Sit comfortably either in a chair or on the floor. Be sure your head is in line with your hips and, if you're seated, that you're not slouching.

- *Inhale* deeply, then *exhale* the air out hard, as if blowing into a balloon. Notice what you feel. If you have the urge to urinate when blowing, your pelvic floor may be weak due to the change in pressure the forced exhalation caused within. Not to worry; you can correct this with focus, awareness, and an intention to do your best work each day.
- Remain relaxed yet aware of your breath moving in and out of your body.
  - To help identify the pelvic floor muscles, I have listed recommendations from anatomy and movement specialist Blandine Calais-Germain (below). Perform these exercises lying down with your knees bent and feet on the ground hip distance apart, fully reclined with legs straight, squatting, or seated. (Standing is too difficult because of the effect of gravity on the body.) Feel each instruction during one inhalation and exhalation as you follow these instructions:
- Feel like you are drawing the tailbone and pubic bone together and keep your awareness on the most exterior muscles between these points.
- Feel like the two bony knobs at the base of the pelvis (the sitting bones) are drawing together.
- Rock the pelvis gently from top to bottom five times.
- Rock the pelvis side to side five times.
- Feel the two lines between the tailbone/public bone and the two sitting bones gently drawing together simultaneously. Feel like you are keeping the pelvic floor flat and not lifting too hard.
- Coordinate this movement with several breath cycles. Exhale while making an S consonant and contract the pelvic floor inwards and up. You can either keep the pelvis still in a neutral position or rock the pelvis back, so the tailbone points toward your bent knees on the exhalation. Inhale fully and relax the pelvic floor completely.[22]

• Hold the pelvic floor contraction and release exercises for these two lengths: a short time (two to five-second contraction) and a long time (seven to ten-second contraction). *Be sure the relaxed time between each contraction is as long as the contraction, so the pelvic floor muscles establish a balance between contracting and expanding.*

As part of your daily regimen, begin with long holds and then finish with short contractions. By giving equal awareness to the two lengths of contractions throughout the day, you can create balance in the elasticity of the muscle fibers that make up the pelvic floor. As Calais-Germain teaches, the short contractions strengthen the muscle cells that contract involuntarily, as in orgasm. By comparison, the long contractions strengthen the muscles making up the bulk and tone of the pelvic floor.[23]

Do *not* inhale deeply while sustaining a pelvic floor contraction because it places too much pressure on the pelvic organs and pelvic floor. This may be contrary to what you may have learned in a prenatal yoga class in which you contracted the pelvic floor on an inhalation and released the pelvic floor on an exhalation. This is because prenatal Kegel exercises focus on connecting the exhalation with releasing the grip of the pelvic floor, which aids in a smoother delivery of the baby. If the pelvic floor is contracted on an exhalation, it will run counter to the mother's energy pushing the baby out on her breath and through a tight muscular region.) You can feel a shallow yet natural breath while sustaining a long contraction. Follow ten long contractions and releases with ten short contractions three to five times a day. An excellent way to remember to do them three times a d right before breakfast, lunch, and dinner. If you want to do them five times a day, add one repetition in the morning after you've visited the toilet and again in the evening before bedtime.

Postural Alignment for Diastasis Recti

In **Part One**, you determined whether you have diastasis recti and to what degree. Here, you will establish the correct alignment of the head, ribs, and pelvis to encourage the two sides of the abdominal sheath to knit together.

- Start by sitting comfortably on the edge of a chair with both feet on the floor. Don't sit back as most chairs have curved back supports that encourage slumping. Feel your sitting bones evenly balanced on the seat of the chair. Feel that your lower belly is as long as your lower back, meaning your tailbone isn't pointing back so far that your lower back is shorter, and your belly is protruding forward. On the other hand, don't let your tailbone point forward with your lower back rounded out and your belly slumped inward. Instead, strongly rise out of your pelvis, with your lower back keeping its natural curve and your lower belly gently engaged from this balanced support. Feel as if this lift of the spine comes because you feel like you're floating through the crown of the head.

- Next, bring your awareness to your ribs. Notice if your lower ribs are vertically aligned with your upper ribs. In other words, don't flare out the lower ribs![24] Instead, place one hand on the lower ribs and the other on the upper ribs by the collar bones. You may feel the lower hand further out than the upper hand if you're sticking out your lower ribs. If that happens, lift your upper ribs up and forward a bit while drawing in your lower ribs and your back. Facilitating this lift requires engaging your deep core muscles. You will feel long in the torso and may even feel a release in the lower and middle back. You may also feel the lower back muscles soften as they come into proper positioning while you discover the appropriate positioning of your pelvis.

- Last, feel the positioning of your head as if you're floating through the crown at the very top of the skull. Feel that the back of your neck is as long as the front of your throat, putting your ears in line with the middle of the tops of your shoulders. When you have optimal posture and a balanced relationship of your pelvis, ribs, and head, you should feel strong throughout your body, yet with a floating sensation.

To sustain the optimal alignment of your ribs, pelvis, and head in daily life, sit upright when you're in the car and don't slump in the bucket seat designs most cars have. Also, resist the temptation to slouch on the sofa while relaxing or nursing the baby. Instead, bring your baby to your breast and roll your shoulders back and down rather than rounding yourself forward.

Now that you've established optimal posture while seated, carry this over to standing.

- As you rise out of the chair, notice what happens to the positioning of your pelvis, ribs, and head. Are they aligned? Now that you know the correct relationship between these parts, you can "build" yourself from the feet up. At the same time, evenly distribute your weight to the front, back, and sides of your feet.
- Next, keep your knees soft (not locked) and align your pelvis such that your lower back feels as long as your lower belly. Then align your ribs appropriately so your lower ribs do not stick out and shorten your middle back.
- Last, float through the crown of your head so your ears are in line with the tops of your shoulders. Make sure the back of your neck and the front of the throat are of equal length to each other.

Birthday Candle Breath

Using your breath awareness and healthy posture, let's do a focused breathing exercise called *Birthday Candle Breath* that tones your transverse abdominus.

- Start sitting in a chair or on a thick folded blanket. Feel your pelvis in a neutral position and your ribs stacked, with the lowest ribs in line with your upper ribs. Place one hand on your upper belly and the other on your collarbones to feel if they are in line with each other.
- *Inhale* into your belly, ribs, and back. Then exhale through your mouth with your lips in the shape of the smallest circle you can comfortably make—about the size of the tip of your pinky finger as if you are saying "who." It's like blowing out a birthday candle three feet away with one focused stream of breath. Do not forcefully push the breath; keep it steady from the beginning of the exhalation to the end.
- Once your lungs feel emptied, pulse the exhalation five times (knowing there's always a small reserve of air in the lungs at the base of an exhalation). You'll feel as if you have a corset on and someone is making the waist a bit smaller with each exhaled puff of air. You will feel an engagement of your lower belly in and up toward the back of your lower ribs. (This is not the same as sucking in your belly. Rather, it's like a zipper effect in which the lower belly is engaged in and upward. It activates the lower part of the transverse abdominus.)
- Fully relax your abdomen on inhalation. Do this series five times.
- Next, *exhale* on an S consonant as if you are a hissing snake (not a forceful snake but a friendly one!). Repeat on three more breaths.

Over time, as the S consonant gets easier, graduate to an F consonant and explore this sound until you feel it is steady and consistent from the beginning of the exhalation to the end. Next, explore a Z consonant as if you are a buzzing bee (not a forceful bee but a friendly one!). Again, keep the sound consistent from the beginning of the exhalation to the end. The more friction the sound has, the more your transverse abdominus hugs in to stabilize while you sustain the quality of the sound from the beginning of the exhalation to the end.

Each day, explore ten *Birthday Candle Breaths* on whichever consonant is appropriate for you. Then add ten pelvic floor contractions and relaxations (PFCR) exercises to the *Birthday Candle Breath*. *Inhale,* relax the pelvic floor; *exhale,* contract the pelvic floor upwardly while exhaling on your consonant. *Inhale,* relax everything, and repeat for as long as you can sustain focus on alignment and breath.

End your movement practice this week with this resting pose.

Rest and Relaxation Pose, *Savasana*

- This pose is traditionally called "Corpse Pose," but I call it *Rest and Relaxation Pose* due to the strong reactions of some people to its actual name. Lie on your mat with your feet hip distance apart and arms alongside the body with the palms up. If your neck feels short or tight while lying on the mat, place a firm folded blanket under your head. Make sure your head and neck align with your spine along the back. If desired, place a blanket over your body to accommodate the slight decrease in body temperature when lying still.
- Breathe here for at least three minutes (better yet, for fifteen minutes!).
    - In this reclined meditation, keep your awareness of your breath and the sensations of your body. Stay relaxed yet softly focused on the sensations within.

Work on creating healthy postural alignment (seated and stand-ing) throughout your daily life as we work together. This is the foundation for all the movement work we do. Let this be part of your intent with this program as you create and nurture habits that support your health and livelihood—now and forever.

Embodied Voice Exploration: Humming to Music

This voice exploration will create awareness of the sensation of your voice through a practice you've done your whole life—hum-ming to music! This time, you will hum to the music you feel *within*. Keep the range of the notes you hum moderate. Think of your vocal range as a house; we want to stay on the main living level. If you go too high, you will be in the attic; if you go too low, you're in the basement of your voice.

Focus on enjoying the vibrations of the voice as you feel them tickling your lips and the bones in your mouth (the hard palate and the teeth).

- Close your eyes or find a soft gaze. Hum on an M consonant and feel the vibration on your lips. Experiment with your lips to notice the change in the quality of the vibration—press your lips hard together and hum, then soften your lips a lot and hum. Next, find the "just right" amount of pressure be-tween your two lips to sense the most vibration at the level that feels good.
- Keep your voice on one pitch or note. Usually saying, "Hello, my name is Mom," and sustaining the M at the end of "Mom" brings you to a pitch comfortable in the conversational speaking range. Feel the vibrations of the M on this one note for different lengths of time—a three-second exhalation, a five-second exhalation.
- Next, feel the vibrations of the M while exploring up and down two or three pitches above your conversational pitch

from before. Focus on keeping the vibrations on your lips and out of your head. Remember, we are exploring the *speaking* voice, not the *singing* voice.

- Continue humming to feel a vibration on your lips. Enjoy the feeling of your voice! Hum as often as possible. Freely hum songs in both your conversational range and your singing range as you practice throughout the week.

Meditation: Notice the Air

This week's meditation is beautiful whenever you want to feel safe, grounded, and connected to your core self and surroundings. Bring your awareness to your breathing and work toward quieting your mind as you begin. You can feed your baby while engaging in this meditation if you like.

- Sit on the edge of a folded blanket in *Easy Pose* to support your pelvis or sit in your favorite chair for feeding your child.
- Feel your breath moving in and out of your nose. Notice the temperature of the air coming in and its warmer temperature going out.
- Stay here for as long as you feed your baby, noticing the breath moving in and out through your nose.

Optional: Read about *non-harming* in **Part Four** and journal what you discover about this practice. I encourage you to continue your exploration of this principle as you move through the program.

Phase One, Week Two

Believe in your path as you tap into the vitality in your practice that's arising. Find the component of your practice that best lifts your spirit and integrates breath, movement, and voice, then let that be the source of energy for other parts of your practice needing a boost. If humming feels good, why not hum through your movement-based practice? Find the synergy among the different elements of the program and keep the faith as you go!

Find the synergy among the different elements of the program and keep the faith as you go!

In **Phase One, Week Two**, continue developing the *Breath-Based Practice, Embodied Voice Exploration,* and *Meditation* from **Phase One, Week One**. This week, we will integrate breath awareness directly into the movement practice.

Moving on the rhythm of your breath takes time to develop. Most people tend to either hold their breath while in motion or move more quickly than their natural breathing rhythm. If you breathe more quickly than how you move, you prevent a true slowing of the mind, which is one of the main purposes of a yoga practice. Matching the mind, breath, and movement brings you to the stillness of the spirit within. Let this be on your mind as you explore the breaths and movements this week.

We will add traditional yoga poses to different movements and body positions to carry over from Week One. In this way, we can practice on the mat, adopting appropriate postures so the six sides of the core can strengthen and establish flexible balance with each other while moving and breathing. Once you can do this on the mat, let's work toward living it "off the mat" daily.

This week's poses create a foundation for your seated practice and release tension in the shoulders, neck, and upper back. Work with loving kindness toward yourself by keeping the range of motion small and building up to more significant movements as you feel ready.

Breath-Based Practice: Continue Finding Awareness

Continue finding awareness through your breath, feeling its movement in and out of your body as you rest and begin your practice each day.

Movement-Based Practice: Adding on to Foundational Practices

1. Come into *Easy Pose or kneeling.*
2. Add *Shoulder/Neck Releases*:

Shoulder/Neck Release: Shoulder Rolls, Gentle Neck Practices

- Sit with your spine long and roll your shoulders up and back on the inhalation.
- Roll them down on an exhalation. Enjoy ten shoulder rolls.
- Bring the right ear toward the right shoulder while keeping the shoulder relaxed down. Breathe several cycles. *Inhale,* float the crown of the head up and *exhale,* bring the left ear to left shoulder. Relax and breathe for several cycles.

Repeat these three practices for as long as you are able while keeping soft attention on your breath and body/mind connection.

3. Explore *Semi-Supine Pelvic Tilts with PFCR:*

Semi-Supine Pelvic Tilts with PFCR

- Lie on your back with knees bent and feet hip distance apart on the floor (a semi-supine position). Feel the length of your spine from the back of your head all the way to your tailbone.

- *Inhale,* rock the tailbone toward the mat while creating more space between your lower back and the floor. *Exhale,* contract the pelvic floor while curling the tailbone up toward the knees and bringing the lower back to the mat.
- *Inhale,* relax the pelvic floor and breathe into the lower abdomen while pointing the tailbone toward the mat. *Exhale,* engage the pelvic floor while tilting your pelvis back so your tailbone points to your knees.

Repeat the pelvic tilts with awareness of pelvic floor contraction and release three to five more times.

Note for C-section mothers: If you feel any pulling near or at your incision site, minimize your range of motion in your mid-to-low back as you tilt the pelvis.

4. Sit in *Staff Pose* while focusing on the equal length and strength of the front body to the back body and the side bodies to each other. Breathe with the *Birthday Candle Breath* for fifteen breaths with pulses, then five exhales on the S consonant.

5. Carry your breath awareness over to the practices making up the Core Foundation: *PFCR* exercises and the *Birthday Candle Breath* for toning the TA and correcting diastasis recti. Continue working with your *Optimal Posture* of sitting and standing for healing diastasis recti.

6. To this, you will add the *Hand Corset* exercise, the fourth item in your Core Foundation practice.

The Hand Corset

- Stand with your back against the wall and slightly bend your knees. Lean the back of the pelvis against the wall.
- Clasp your hands around your ribs with the fingers pointing toward each other. Press your hands toward each other as if

interweaving the muscle fibers of the two sides of the abdomen. Your hands will draw together like a corset.

• Sustain this gentle, yet firm, compression for a few breaths. Then move along the length of the abdomen from the lower ribs to the pelvis similarly.

If you incorporate this exercise with postural alignment and optimal breathing, you can encourage the muscles of the rectus abdominus to knit back together.

7. End your movement practice with five minutes of *Rest and Relaxation Pose*.

Embodied Voice Exploration: Musical Humming and Tapping

• Continue to *Hum to Feel Music*, playing with different rhythms and pitches.
• Add musical tapping (feeling the sounds D, T, B, P, G, K as musical instruments) to your exploration. Take your time to feel the sensations of each. They are each unique.
• Play with the parts of the tongue that create these tapped sounds and enjoy the rhythms you create.

Meditation: Notice the Air

Continue to *Notice the Air* as you sit and breathe for five minutes.

Phase Two

For most people, (deep insight into complete absorption of the heart-mind) is preceded by faith, vitality, strong memory, samadhi, then deep insight.
Yoga Sutra 1.20

By now, you have had faith that you are on the right path to wellness and integration in body, mind, voice, and spirit. You are finding vitality in your practice and hopefully creating a bodymind memory of what feels best for you. Let your bodymind lead the way as you explore these practices, and you will naturally remember what is optimal for you.

We will carry our awareness of sensation in our foundational practices into sustaining movements that bring us more dynamic expression. Your *Movement-Based Practice* will strengthen your core and support your postural alignment on and off the mat. Your *Breath-Based Practice* will deepen your awareness of your breathing rhythm and the inner space within. Your *Embodied Voice Practice* carries musical humming into sustained consonants for feeling musicality in your speaking voice. Arthur Lessac asks if you felt like you were singing when you were speaking.[25] If you don't, this is the time to feel the same spiritual connection to your speaking voice as you do to your singing voice. It's the same voice—it's you! Finally, your *Meditation Practice* extends your awareness of your breath to its dynamics as it moves in and out of you.

Community Prompt

Go to the supermarket and purposefully work toward engaging with other people. Make eye contact. Smile. If you see a parent buying a particular baby product, ask how they like it and initiate a short conversation. Perhaps share information about a product you enjoy and why. If no one is shopping the baby aisle that day, ask the store manager about a community bulletin board and search for new mom meet-up groups. If there aren't any, do you feel inspired to start one?

Phase Two, Week One

Breath-Based Practice: Even Ratio Breath, *Sama Vritti Pranayama*

- Lie back comfortably with knees bent and feet on the floor. Feel your spine on the mat with your pelvis, ribs, shoulders, and head in line with each other. Breathe comfortably.
- *Inhale* on a count of three, hold it softly for a count of three, *exhale* on a count of three, then keep your breath out for three seconds before your next inhalation. This creates an equal ratio of breath for all four stages of breathing: inhalation, being filled with breath, exhalation, being empty of breath.
- Continue with the even ratio breathing for ten breath cycles. Adjust the count for what feels comfortable, whether two seconds or five seconds.

Movement-Based Practice: Feel Length in the Spine

1. Sit comfortably in *Easy Pose* or kneeling and enjoy the neck release and ten shoulder rolls backward on the rhythm of the breath (*inhale*, shoulders up; *exhale*, roll them back and down).
2. Add *Eagle Arms:*

Eagle Arms, *Garudasana*

- Inhale your arms to shoulder height like you are making the letter T, exhale, and bring the arms in front with the right above the left.
- Bend your elbows and intertwine your lower arms with each other. (Optional: If comfortable, cross your wrists and touch your palms.)
- Breathe several cycles. *Inhale*, uncross your arms, and return to shoulder height. *Exhale* the arms to the front of the body, and bring the left arm above the right, bending the elbows as before (or cross at the wrists, if appropriate). Breathe several breaths before releasing your arms.
- Rest your hands on your thighs. Breathe and notice openness in your shoulders and neck.

3. Explore *Six Directions for the Spine:*

Six Directions for the Spine

- Sit in *Easy Pose* on one or two folded blankets to prop the sitting bones at the base of the pelvis or kneel. Lengthen the spine. *Inhale* the arms up and *exhale* while placing your right hand on the floor and reaching the left arm overhead for a **side bend**.
- Breathe into your left ribs. *Inhale* both arms up while coming back to a neutral spine. *Exhale* your left hand to the floor while reaching your right arm overhead for a **side bend**. Breathe into your right ribs. *Inhale* both arms up while returning to a neutral spine. *Exhale* and relax both arms down.
- *Inhale* both arms up and twist to the right while keeping a **twist** mainly in the upper back. *Exhale* both arms down and make contact with the floor and right thigh. *Inhale*, lengthen the spine; *exhale*, engage with the twist.

- *Inhale* both arms up and *exhale* while **twisting** to the left. Make contact with the floor and left thigh. Breathe. *Inhale* both arms up to return to a neutral spine. *Exhale* and relax. Keep the twist in the upper-to-mid back.

Note for C-section mothers: Minimize your range of motion in the twists if you feel any pulling near or at your incision site.

- As you *inhale* and roll your shoulders back, bring your hands behind and engage your shoulder blades down your back while broadening your chest. Look up while lengthening your throat for a **back bend**. *Exhale* and breathe here.
- *Inhale*, bring the shoulders forward to neutral, then rest your hands on your thighs. *Inhale* both arms up and *exhale* while rounding your shoulders **forward** to expand your upper back. Do not collapse the ribs into the pelvis. Rather, stay long in the front of the spine without collapsing forward. Breathe. *Inhale* both arms up, *exhale*, and relax with your hands on your thighs.

4. Add *Hero Pose:*

Hero Pose, *Virasana*

- Come onto your shins in a kneeling position.
- Fold the blanket so it is a rectangular shape, then trifold the blanket so it becomes a firm bolster (or use a bolster if you have one). Place the length of the blanket on your mat.
- Roll the flesh of your calves towards the sides of your mat and sit on the edge of your folded blanket or bolster. The higher you prop your pelvis, the more space you can create in the knees if you feel your knees are tense. If this is the case, roll the edge of the blanket tri-fold one time over and sit.

- Align the soles of your feet so all five toes equally touch the mat. Sit here with optimal rib-to-pelvis alignment and breathe five to eight breaths. When finished, remove your prop from your yoga mat.

5. Add *Table Pose, Cow Pose, Cat Pose*

Table Pose (*Bharmanasana*), Cow Pose (*Bitilasana*), Cat Pose (*Marjariasana*)

- *Table Pose:* Come onto all four, hands under your shoulders and knees under your hips. Keep your elbows slightly soft so the elbow creases face each other and not forward. Find length in the spine, keeping your lower ribs engaged inward to stay long in the front of the torso.
- *Cow Pose:* Inhale the breastbone forward and up while keeping the lower back as neutral and long as possible. Look up if it feels nice for the neck. We are concentrating the backbend in this pose in the upper back.
- *Cat Pose:* Exhale while rounding your upper back, spreading your shoulder blades apart, and engaging your navel toward your spine to feel length in y lower belly and lower back. Do not suck in your belly; instead, seek to feel a deep core engagement.
- Repeat the movements from *Cow Pose* to *Cat Pose* three to five times. Work slowly. To add PFCR, inhale and relax the pelvic floor on *Cow Pose*, then exhale and contract on *Cat Pose*. To add extra transverse abdominus toning, include the *Birthday Candle Breath*.

6. Explore *Bird Dog Pose:*

Bird Dog Pose, *Dandayamana Bharmanasana*

- Engage your lower ribs toward the spine.
- From *Table Pose*, extend your right arm forward parallel to the floor while extending the left leg back. Let your toes touch the mat or lift your leg while rolling your inner thigh down.
- Keep your lower ribs engaged toward the spine. Also, keep your pelvis balanced.
- Breathe three to five breaths before returning to *Table Pose*. Repeat on the other side. Repeat this movement sequence three to five times.

7. Explore *Extended Child's Pose:*

Extended Child's Pose, *Balasana*

- Kneel with your thighs either aligned with each other or open wide to make room for abdominal flesh. Kneeling with the thighs together will give a nice abdominal toning.
- Extend your arms and engage your palms into the mat. Rest your forehead on the mat or a yoga block and rest your hips toward your heels. (If your hips don't comfortably rest on your heels, sit on a wide yoga block between the shins or ankles. If your forehead doesn't touch the floor, you may rest your forehead on a yoga block.)
- Breathe easily and feel your back expanding with each breath.

8. Begin your work reviewing the Core Foundation: *Pelvic Floor Contraction and Release* (PFCR) exercises while lying on your back with your knees bent, sitting upright, and finding *Optimal Postural Alignment* of pelvis, ribs, and head, the *Hand Corset*, and the *Birthday Candle Breath* with the exhalation on the S consonant.

9. Move to *Legs Up the Wall Pose:*

Legs Up the Wall Pose, *Viparita Karani*

- Get a firm folded blanket and fold it into a quarter fold and then a trifold so it's about one foot wide.
- Place the blanket six to eight inches away from the base-board of a wall clear from framed art or other obstacles. The distance of the blanket from the baseboard depends on the length of your legs and flexibility in your hips and lower back.
- Sit on the short edge of the blanket and pivot back to place the legs up the wall while using your hands to help you lie back. You can adjustments as needed to align your legs up the wall and also align your spine with your pelvis.
- Lay your arms out like a T with palms facing up. Rest there for several minutes.
- Come down, curl your knees into your chest, and roll onto your right side. You can use your hands to push yourself up slowly.

10. Enjoy *Rest and Relaxation Pose* for three to five minutes.

Embodied Voice Exploration: M and N Consonants

Phase Two adds to the sensations of humming by carrying it into sustained consonants. "Sustained" means humming on the length of a natural exhalation. As you sustain consonants, play with feeling the same quality of the sound from the beginning to the end of the word. You're working against the voice trailing off at the end of the word or going into a crackling sound at the end, also known as "vocal fry."

- Begin by humming to feel vibration on your lips. Enjoy the musicality of your voice. Now feel the M in words that end with M while sustaining it a second or two longer than you normally would. This is not an invitation to be loud or force-ful with the sound. Rather, it's to explore duration (the length of time you hum the sound) in speaking. This plays with the rhythm and tempo of the humming.

- Explore these words, then find your own: **mom, him, same, seem, flame, momentum, came, postpartum.**
- Feel the M when it ends a syllable and even when it's in the middle of a word that doesn't end with M. Notice the fun changes in tempo and musicality when sustaining the M for a moment longer than the other consonants. Feel it in these words, then find your own: **symptom, amplitude, member-ship, exclaim, kingdom.**
- Start with musical humming on an M. Next, shift the hum to an N and feel the vibrations of the N consonant. Then feel the connection between the tip of the tongue as it softly engages with the gum ridge at the apex of your upper front teeth. Let the rest of your tongue relax and your lips rest forward as if you're about to softly kiss your baby.
- Now hum on the N through a simple song and notice the quality of its vibration. Does the vibration waft into the sinus cavity or even the front of the forehead? Feel the N on an exhalation of different lengths, just as you did with the M. Now feel the N on different pitches of the speaking voice while keeping the range small. Don't rush it; you have a lot to feel and notice on only three or four pitches. Because people naturally go up in pitch when asking a question, try placing a question mark behind each word in the list and notice how that feels.
- Now feel the N in words that end with an N while sustaining its sound as if for emphasis. Notice if you're able to explore emphasis without pushing your voice or getting louder. This becomes an important skill as your child grows and you need to stress important lessons without force or violence in your voice.

- Explore these words, then find your own: **mine, shine, town, clean, vibration, down, invitation, temptation.**

Meditation: Deepening Awareness of Breath

Either kneel, sit in *Easy Pose,* or lie back in *Rest and Relaxation Pose.* Feel the sensation of your breath as it comes in through your nose. Notice its cool temperature. Feel the pathway the breath takes inwardly—how it expands parts of the body, including your chest, belly, sides, and back. As you *exhale,* feel it leave the body, allowing it to return to its relaxed state. Notice the temperature is a bit warmer on the exhalation. Continue feeling the breath, its temperature, and its pathway in and out of your body for five minutes.

Optional: Read about *truthfulness* in **Part Four** and journal what you discover about this practice. Continue your exploration of this principle as you move through the program.

Phase Two, Week Two

Before you begin your practices this week, take time to look inward and discover your intention for practice every time you come onto the mat. Your intention becomes a reminder of why you're taking this path today. It's a touchstone for your faith in your spiritual life and connection to your true self. Honor it. Feel your breath. Begin.

Breath-Based Practice: Even Ratio Breath

- Continue to explore the *Even Ratio Breath* lying on the ground in a semi-supine position.
- Add one second to the length of each part of the breath cycle.

Movement-Based Practice: Gathering Strength

This week, we add strengthening exercises to tone the muscles that surround your pelvis and support the pelvic floor: the inner and outer thigh muscles (adductors and abductors).

1. Begin your work reviewing the core foundations: *Pelvic Floor Contraction and Relaxation* (PFCR) exercises while lying on your back with your knees bent or by sitting upright and finding *Optimal Postural Alignment* of the pelvis, ribs, and head, the *Hand Corset*, and the *Birthday Candle Breath* with the exhalation on the S consonant.
2. Move to *Table Pose* and flow from *Cow Pose* to *Cat Pose* on the rhythm of your breath while also engaging Feel 10 of these flows as you *inhale* in *Cow Pose* (release pelvic floor) and *exhale* in *Cat Pose* (contract pelvic floor).
3. Move to *Locust Pose:*

Locust Pose, *Salabhasana*

- Fold a blanket about one-foot wide and place it below your breast line on the middle ribs if you are nursing.
- Lie on your belly. The blanket will elevate your breasts off the floor to minimize pressure on your mammary glands. (If you feel tender under your pubic bone, especially if you've had a C-section, you may want a second blanket folded wide and thin placed underneath your hips.)
- As you lie on your belly, align your feet, hips, ribs, and head. Then place your arms alongside your body and put your feet together. *Inhale*, lengthen your spine; *exhale*, raise your chest off the floor and lengthen through your hands with the palms facing your thighs. Keep your feet on the floor and rest for one or two breaths. Repeat two or three more times.

If your shoulders don't feel tight, you can explore this pose with your arms out ahead of you and palms facing each other. If it feels safe for your lower back (no lower back or pelvis pain on the first option) on the exhalation, you may lift your legs, bringing the toes only one or two inches off the floor. To keep length in your lower back, engage your pubic bone downward and forward as if it is scooping toward your nose.

4. Explore *Clamshells, Inner/Outer Thigh Lift:*

Clamshells, Inner/Outer Thigh Lift

- Lie on your right side with your hips flexed and legs bent comfortably. Your knees are stacked, feet are together, and you are resting on your right forearm. Align your feet with your pelvis and engage the lower ribs towards the spine.
- Open your legs while keeping your toes touching. You will feel this action outside the hip, and your legs will open and close like a clamshell.
- Repeat this motion ten times while working slowly with the rhythm of your breath.
- Once you have completed the ten *Clamshells*, straighten your right leg, and lay your left knee over it on the floor. Alternatively, bend your left knee and place your left foot on the floor in front of your right thigh—whichever is more comfortable for you.
- *Inhale*, extend through the heel.
- *Exhale*, lift the right leg up for *Inner Thigh Lifts*. Pulse it up and down on the breath ten times. You want to keep the movement small and controlled to target your adductors (inner thighs).
- Once you have completed the *Inner Thigh Lift*, straighten your left leg, and lay it on top of your right leg. Roll the left thigh inward so your left toes point toward the floor.

- Lift your left leg ten times for *Outer Thigh Lifts.* Keep the movement small and controlled; there is no need to lift the leg more than hip height. Repeat the outer thigh lift nine more times.
- Repeat the series lying on your left side.

5. Explore *Floor Angels:*

Floor Angels[26]

- Lie with a bolster or a folded blanket along your spine and a yoga block beneath your head to encourage your lower ribs to rest.
- *Inhale,* bringing both arms up toward each other overhead while keeping them on the floor.
- *Exhale,* bringing the arms back down the same pathway to your sides—as if you're making snow angels on the floor. Focus on feeling the lower ribs rest down, lengthening the sides of the body, and isolating the movements of the shoulders from movements of the chest and ribs. Do five to ten with easy, focused breaths.
- Remove the bolster under your back and lie on your back.

6. Move into *Semi-Supine Toe Taps:*

Semi-Supine Toe Taps

- Lie on your back with your knees bent about 90 degrees and feet hip distance apart on the floor.
- Feel the length of your spine from the back of your head to the tailbone, then place both hands on the lower belly between your navel and pubic bone. *Inhale* into your lower belly.

- *Exhale,* lifting the right foot and tap the toe to the floor about four inches farther out, then bring it back to its starting position. *Inhale* into the lower belly with feet neutral.
- *Exhale,* lifting the left foot and tap the toe to the floor about four inches farther out, then bring it back to the starting position.
- Repeat for either side four to six more times. Use the hands on the lower belly to feel the movement initiating from the lower belly (transverse abdominus) and not from the hip flexor at the top of the thigh where it meets the hip. Move slowly and on the rhythm of the breath.

7. Roll onto your side and sit on the edge of a folded blanket for *Staff Pose.* Do ten *Birthday Candle Breaths* here.

8. Come into *Extended Child's Pose* for ten natural breaths.

9. Come to *Rest and Relaxation Pose* on your back for three to five minutes.

Note for C-section mothers: If you feel any pulling near or at your incision site, minimize your range of motion regarding how high you lift your leg. The more of a bend you have in your knee and the closer your foot is to your hips, the easier the movement will be. Start small and work toward achieving a larger range of motion over time.

Embodied Voice Exploration: V and Z Consonants

- Place your upper front teeth on your lower lip where the wet, inner part meets the dry, outer lip. Engage your lips softly forward as if you're about to kiss your baby and hum. Find your way to a V. It will feel rich and buzzy. Exhale and vocalize into this contact point without forcing the sound. Over time, you will find your way to a true V sound. When you do, let go of the breathy F that may appear.

- Once you find the V, explore going up and down in pitch. You will feel an engagement with the transverse abdominus. After humming on the V and feeling the consistency of its quality of vibration on the pitches explored so far, begin to feel it in words that end in V: **love, live, dove, strive, improve, and positive.** Feel it as it ends syllables: **driveway, positively, tentatively.** Can you feel the same quality V in the middle of words as you feel on its own or at the end of words?

- Now find a rich, buzzy Z. Sometimes it's fun to pretend a pen is a bumblebee and create its buzz while it flies. (Childlike play always frees the voice in some way.) Once you feel the Z optimally, sustain it on one note. Feel the swirling rumble at the front of the mouth. Notice how to increase its vitality the more you feel the forward-moving action of the lips as if you're about to kiss your baby.

- Over time, the Z will feel full of vibration and not have any hints of the S with it. Once you feel the Z, explore it up and down a few pitches, keeping it in the speaking voice range. Can you sustain the same quality vibration on the different pitches? The more you can, the more you free your vocal life and give yourself more expressive possibilities to be dynamic in your speaking voice without resorting to volume or force to be heard or to stress a point.

- Now feel the Z as it ends words or syllables: **cheers, years, his, hers, because, wisdom, size, sympathize, sizzling, amazed.**

- Continue in this progression with the following consonant sounds until you feel an appreciation for their true beauty and musicality: TH (as in **soothe, breathe**), ZH (as in **garage, mirage**), L (as in **doll, wolf**), and NG (as in **sing, ink**).

Meditation: Deepening Awareness of Breath

Either *kneel*, sit in *Easy Pose* or *Hero Pose*, or lie back in *Rest and Relaxation Pose*. Feel the sensation of your breath as it comes in through your nose. Notice its cool temperature. Feel the path the breath takes inwardly—how it expands parts of the body, including your chest, belly, sides, and back. Feel it leave as you exhale, and your body returns to its relaxed state. Notice the temperature is a bit warmer on the exhalation than on the inhalation. Continue feeling the breath—its temperature and its pathway in and out of the body for five minutes.

Phase Three

For most people, (deep insight into complete absorption of the heart-mind) is preceded by faith, vitality, strong memory, samadhi, then deep insight.
Yoga Sutra 1.20

You have faith in your practice and, most importantly, faith in yourself. You know why this work is important because you are reminded of it every time you see your baby's gorgeous face. The more you take care of yourself, the better you care for your baby. Your mutual love and adoration synergize with the vitality you have created in your practice and livelihood. Your bodymind knows what is best, and you may be getting a glimpse of samadhi—the bliss that comes from a true integration with the Divine spirit inside you and all around you.

Don't stay attached to that feeling—it's always there for you so there is no need to grasp it. Stay present and grounded with your path and enjoy *samadhi* (bliss) whenever it comes. Find gratitude for it.

By now, you are feeling stronger and more connected in body, mind, voice, and spirit. Your energy levels are improving through the subtle harnessing of core strength, vocal resonance, and meditation. In **Phase Three**, we'll continue strengthening your core and also explore lengthening your spine and side bodies in standing postures and gentle twists.

Continue reviewing the practices in **Phase One** to establish dynamic and flexible muscle tone in the pelvic floor and transverse abdominus and keep your pelvis/ribs/head postural alignment within your ongoing awareness. You will feel freer to move more dynamically the more you keep these components of yourself at the forefront of your mind. Over time, your bodymind will sustain this stability and you will be able to free your energy to another part of your wellness path.

The *Breath-Based Practice* is a popularly used breath control practice used in yoga due to its ability to focus the mind inwardly while developing subtle heat in the body if employed throughout the movement practice. It is also an enjoyable, meditative practice on its own. Try it both ways and discover what you prefer.

The *Movement-Based Practices* will lengthen and strengthen more of the core, including the inner and outer oblique muscles. Remember to feel length in the spine for the twists and feel both sides of the waist as equal in length to each other as you move from one pose to the next, even the side bends.

The *Embodied Voice Practices* move from humming into tapping to feeling rhythm in your speech. You will complete this phase by exploring vocal tone such that you feel the subtle power of your voice without any pushing or force. The *Meditation Practice* will harness your focus more directly on the breath and its movement in the body.

Community Prompt

Find the events calendar for your local library and search for Storytime with Children. These events are fun and focused on kids gaining time together and moms interacting. Engage in conversation with another mom and schedule an additional meet-up time with her at the library. Libraries make wonderful spaces for social time. They are climate-controlled, have ample seating, and allow you to bring your food and drinks. As your child gets older, you can also place out a stack of board books for them to sort through while you connect with a friend in a seating area.

Phase Three, Week One

Breath-Based Practice: Victorious Breath

This breath practice is one of the most popular in yoga because it can draw your focus inward. Keep the contraction in the voice small, so the sound that comes is audible only to you.

Victorious Breath, *Ujjayi*

- *Kneel*, sit in *Hero Pose* or *Easy Pose* and feel long in the spine through the crown of the head. *Inhale* comfortably. *Exhale* while *slightly* constricting the back of the throat as if fogging a mirror with your breath. Sustain this slight constriction while inhaling and exhaling. This breath should sound like ocean waves ebbing and flowing on the shore and should only be audible to you.
- Sustain *Victorious Breath* throughout your yoga practice as an inward point of concentration, if desired. Alternately, feel *Victorious Breath* whenever you want to sit and tune inward on the breath when you feel energetically scattered throughout the day.
- Release *Victorious Breath* and return to natural breathing for daily life. *Victorious Breath* can calm anxiety, increase oxygen flow in the blood, and gently heat the body from within.

Movement-Based Practice: Adding Awareness of the Side Body

1. Begin in a semi-supine position and explore pelvic tilts with *PFCR* for ten to fifteen breath cycles.
2. Rest for a breath, then explore *Semi-Supine Toe Taps* while bringing your foot a little farther away from your hips. Explore ten taps with each leg as you breathe. Your leg will be

a little less bent than when you started these in **Phase Two**. Keep your lower back long and grounded to engage the core as you move.

3. Roll onto your side and do ten of each of the *Clamshells, Inner Thigh Lift,* and *Outer Thigh Lift* exercises.

4. Repeat on your other side. Roll onto your belly and explore *Locust Pose* while holding the pose for three to five breaths. Complete three elevations in *Locust Pose.*

5. Come back to *Extended Child's Pose* for five breaths. Move back onto your right side.

6. Add *Modified Side Plank:*

Modified Side Plank, *Vasisthasana*

- Keep your lower ribs engaged in and find equal length in both sides of the waist.
- Rest on your right side with your legs in line with your torso. Place a small bend in the knees. Align the elbow under the shoulder and rest on the right forearm with the palm down and perpendicular to the shoulder. Engage the shoulder blades down the back.
- *Inhale*, feeling the ribs align with the pelvis without flaring out your lower ribs.
- *Exhale*, grounding through the right forearm and hand while lifting your hips. Stabilize through the grounded knee on the mat.
- Place your left hand either on the hip or extend it up so both upper arms are in a straight line.
- Breathe five to eight breaths, then come down. Rest for a moment, then repeat once or twice more.
- Roll onto your left side and repeat the series.

7. Add *Supine Crescent Stretch:*

Supine Crescent Stretch

- Lie on your back with your legs straight and arms alongside the body. Rest and breathe.
- *Inhale* your arms overhead and bring your hands together.
- *Exhale*, reaching your hands to the upper right corner of the mat and then walking the heels of your feet to the lower right corner of the mat.
- Stay here or cross the left ankle over the right to lengthen a little more on the left side of your body without twisting it.
- Breathe into your ribs for five to ten breaths. *Inhale*, grounding into the mat and uncross the ankles (if crossed). *Exhale*, walking your heels to the lower left corner of the mat, and then reach your hands to the upper left corner of the mat. If you like, cross the right ankle over the left without twisting the spine too much.
- Breathe into your ribs for five to ten breaths. *Inhale*, grounding deeply. *Exhale*, walking the heels of your feet to the center, with your hands to the center, releasing your arms alongside your body.

8. Add *Gate Pose:*

Gate Pose, *Parighasana*

- *Kneel* with optimal ribs-to-pelvis alignment. If you feel pressure in your knees, kneel on a folded blanket.
- Hold a yoga block in your right hand and extend your right leg out and the sole of your foot on the floor (toes pointing forward and outer arch of the foot parallel to the short side of your yoga mat). You can extend the leg and point the toes up while balancing on the heel. Do whichever option feels more comfortable to you.
- Feel length in both sides of your waist, then *inhale.*

- *Exhale*, extend your right hand with the block down, feeling the right side of your waist contract as it did in *Modified Side Plank* to support the weight of the spine.
- Reach the left hand up toward the ceiling. Let your chest stay open with your collarbones wide. If extending the left arm is too difficult to balance, place your hand on the right hip. Breathe here for five breaths.
- *Inhale* to return to kneeling and repeat for the other side with the left leg extended.

9. Add *Extended Puppy Dog Pose:*

Extended Puppy Dog Pose

- Start in *Extended Child's Pose* with your hands grounded on the mat and sitting back on your heels. Feel the length of your spine.
- *Inhale* into your back ribs.
- *Exhale* and lift your hips with your tailbone pointing to the top of the wall behind you while keeping your knees bent at least 90 degrees.

This pose is about lengthening your spine, not stretching the backs of your legs, so keep your lower ribs engaged toward the spine and not flaring out. After regular practice, if you feel strong in the shoulders and back and *do not have a flaring out of the ribs*, explore straightening the legs into a fuller expression of *Downward Facing Dog (Adho Mukha Svanasana)*.

10. Add *Mountain Pose:*

Mountain Pose, *Tadasana*

- Stand with your feet a couple of inches apart.

- Slowly rock from heel to toe to feel the inner and outer arches of the feet.
- Spread your toes to feel the arch beneath the ball of the foot. Find a comfortable balance between heel-to-toe and the toe spread.
- Lift your spine by feeling a sense of floating through the crown of your head. Keep your ribs stacked above your pelvis. Feel length in both sides of your waist. Feel as if you have an "air pillow" behind your kneecaps to engage them up the front of your thigh while keeping the backs of your knees soft.
- Feel grounded and strong while breathing into your abdomen, sides, and back.

11. Add *Half Sun Salutations:*

Half Sun Salutations

Keep these salutations gentle, and only do them if you can raise your arms overhead without flaring out your lower ribs. Keep your knees bent for standing forward folds so you don't strain your lower back.

- Begin in *Mountain Pose* with two blocks in front of your feet.
- *Inhale* your arms up by lifting them straight in front of you and up for *Tall Mountain Pose.* Resist flaring your ribs and sustain optimal rib-to-pelvis alignment.
- *Exhale*, bending your knees a lot and folding at the hips—not at the waist—to bring your chest toward your thighs.
- Place your hands on your yoga blocks. *Inhale*, pressing your hands into the blocks to extend the spine and bring the shoulder blades down the back. Come to a feeling of a flat back.
- *Exhale*, bringing your chest and thighs toward each other again.
- *Inhale*, grounding through the feet as you keep your knees soft and rise to *Tall Mountain Pose.*

- *Exhale*, moving your arms down to *Mountain Pose*.
- Repeat two more times.

Note for C-section mothers: If you feel any pulling on or near your incision site, place your yoga blocks on the tall setting or use the seat or back of a chair to place your hands for the standing forward fold and extended standing forward fold ("flat back").

12. Add *Reclined Twist*:

Reclined Twist, *Jathara Parivartanasana*

- Lie on your back with knees bent and together and feet together. Have a blanket folded like a bolster next to your right buttock.
- Bring your arms out like a T.
- *Inhale,* lifting your shins so they are parallel to the ceiling.
- Place a yoga block on the skinny setting between your knees or lower thigh. *Exhale,* feeling your core activate as you slowly move your knees to the right while slightly squeezing the block. Feel grounded through your hands and upper back. (It's okay if the shoulder blade opposite your knees is off the mat. Don't force it to stay on the mat.) Your thighs should be resting on the blanket-bolster to ease pressure in the pelvis.
- Relax and breathe. Soften into the twist and hold.
- After five to ten breaths, *inhale* the shins back up.
- Slide the bolster-blanket to the left buttock. *Exhale,* engage the core, and bring the knees with the block to the left. Relax and breathe for five to ten breaths.
- *Inhale* your shins back up one at a time and *exhale* the feet to the mat hip-distance apart.
- Release the block.

13. Relax in *Rest and Relaxation Pose* for five to ten minutes.

Embodied Voice Exploration: B/P, D/T, G/K Consonants

In addition to beautiful humming sounds, we have tapped sounds that add rhythm to our language and a sparkling texture to how we feel our speech. Just like the mallet of a drum, the tapped consonants have a "spring-away" action. The drummer doesn't let the mallet thud on the drum's skin; it bounces back. Otherwise, the sounds become heavy and cumbersome. Instead, we want to re-capture the jazzy, lightness of tapped consonants as music.

- Start by humming on an M. Notice where you feel the vibration on your lips. Now feel a small explosive action on this point and find a B.
- Tap like you tap a drum, feeling the point of connection as well as the point of the "spring-away" of the lips. For fun, tap it on different pitches in your speaking vocal range. Feel it as you explore: **crib, job, doorknob, subject, absorb, abdomen, cobweb, suburb.**
- Continue tapping on the B and then stop vocalizing while you continue tapping. Notice the soft beauty of the P, a sound that is present without any need to push. Feel it in: **pump, pop, asleep, lollipop, strap, clasp, wipe, stomp.**
- Feel an N and hum on it. Notice the tip of the tongue gently pressing on the upper gum ridge.
- Tap there with the "spring-away" action and feel a D consonant. Play it with joy and enjoy the quality of the vocal vibration each time. Feel it as you explore: **did, dad, feed, fooled, led, squeezed, stampede, amplitude.** Now tap on the D and feel it without your voice.
- Notice the beautiful crisp nature of the T. Feel the T without any push—enjoy its potent lightness. Now feel the T in: **cat, bait, late, mate, object, elephant, faint, waft.**
- Feel the word "sing" and notice the contact of the back of the tongue at the back of the mouth where the hard palate meets

the soft palate. Relax the rest of the tongue and sustain this contact point with the forward-moving action of the lips and cheeks. This is the NG consonant sound felt in: **hang, sing, ink, bring, teething, juncture.**

- Now, tap the back of the tongue on this contact point and feel the G consonant. Sustain the forward-moving action of the lips and cheeks so you don't swallow the sound; keep it moving forward. Feel the G in: **dig, big, zigzag, leg, brag, log, diaper bag, jog.**
- Now tap the G and make it unvoiced and feel the crisp tap of the K consonant. There's no need to push out the sound; if you feel it, others will hear it. Tap the K for fun. Now feel it in: **make, shake, cake, music, drink, cowlick, back, unpack.**

Meditation: Counting with the Breath

Notice how long it takes to have a relaxed inhalation. Softly hold your breath until your body and mind are satisfied and then *exhale* while adding one or two more counts. Let your lungs remain still for a moment before inhaling and repeating. If you *inhale* on a count of four, you will *exhale* on a count of six. Continue this counting rhythm for anywhere from three to five minutes.

Optional: Read about *non-stealing* in **Part Four** and journal what you discover about this practice. I encourage you to continue your exploration of this principle as you move through the program.

Phase Three, Week Two

Tap more deeply into your spiritual connection to your values and what you *know in your soul* is best for you. Dive inward and know that all that you need to feel well in this world resides within.

Your breath is the road that takes you there. Follow it and its meandering ways. You'll come into your true Divine self and feel beauty.

Breath-Based Practice: Victorious Breath

Continue exploring the subtleties of *Victorious Breath* such that you feel and hear it, but someone two or three feet away from you does not. You do not want to force the exhalation as that will bring tension in the throat. Instead, feel the slight constriction that brings warmth and an internal point of focus to your practice.

Movement-Based Practice: Strengthening the Hips

1. Start with ten to fifteen *Semi-Supine Toe Taps* while bringing your foot a little farther away from your hips. Your leg will be a little less bent than when you started these in **Phase Two**. Keep your lower back long and grounded to engage your core as you move.
2. Roll onto your side and do ten of each of the *Clamshells, Inner Thigh Lift,* and *Outer Thigh Lift* exercises.
3. Move into *Modified Side Plank* for ten breaths.
4. Repeat the *Clamshells, Inner Thigh Lift, Outer Thigh Lift,* and *Modified Side Plank* on your other side.
5. Roll onto your belly and explore the *Locust Pose,* holding it for three to five breaths. Complete three elevations in *Locust Pose.*
6. Press back into *Extended Child's Pose* for two to three breaths.
7. Move onto your hands and knees and explore five extensions in *Bird Dog Pose* on each side while feeling your deep core connections supporting you.
8. Come to standing and move through three *Half Sun Salutations.*
9. Add *Goddess Pose:*

Goddess Pose, *Utkata Konasana*

- Begin in *Mountain Pose* at the center of the mat, facing the long side of the mat.
- Step your feet wide, then shorten your stride by about 30% to preserve the ligaments of the pelvis.

- Pivot on your heels and point the balls of your feet to the corners of the long side of the yoga mat. Keep your hands on your hips and squat downwards while lining up your ribs with your pelvis.
- Bring your arms up and engage your shoulder blades down your back while bending your elbows, making your arms resemble a goal post. Again, resist flaring out your lower ribs. Breathe here for five breaths.
- *Inhale*, grounding through the feet, and rise.
- Lower your arms and step the feet together a few inches at a time returning to *Mountain Pose*.

9. Come to kneeling with a blanket folded like a bolster and enjoy ten shoulder and neck releases before coming into *Rest and Relaxation Pose*. You may take *Rest and Relaxation* in the kneeling position so it's like a seated meditation.

Embodied Voice Exploration: Double Rhythm

Continue playing with the rhythm of the tapped consonants B, P, D, T, G, and K. Explore the double rhythm they provide when they appear together. Play both for clarity, variety, and musicality: KT (**act, sacked**), GD (**begged, bagged**), PT (**apt, clamped**), and BD (**rubbed, sobbed**). Feel each consonant clearly while honoring them as a coupled rhythm.

Meditation: Counting with the Breath

Notice how long it takes to have a relaxed inhalation. Softly hold your breath until your body and mind are satisfied and then *exhale* while adding one or two more counts. Let your lungs remain still for a moment before inhaling and repeating. If you *inhale* on a count of four, you will *exhale* on a count of six. Continue this counting rhythm for anywhere from four to six minutes.

Phase Three, Week Three

Stay curious about yourself as you practice. There is always so much to discover. Let yourself be amazed by what you find.

Breath-Based Practice: Victorious Breath
Continue feeling the *Victorious Breath* and let it become a point of meditation for your movement-based practice.

Movement-Based Practice: Adding Twists That Lengthen and Release the Spine and Side Body

1. Review the *Core Foundation* from **Phase One**: *PFCR, Postural Alignment for Healing Diastasis Recti, Hand Corset, Birthday Candle Breath* on a Z consonant exhalation.
2. Move into *Table Pose* and explore *Cow Pose* and *Cat Pose* with PFCR for ten cycles.
3. Move into *Extended Puppy Dog Pose* to lengthen the spine for five breaths.
4. Come to *Mountain Pose* and feel grounded through the feet.
5. Add *Standing Crescent Stretch*:

Standing Crescent Stretch

- Stand with your back against the wall and your weight equally distributed on your feet. Feel tall, like you are floating through the crown of the head without letting the lower ribs flare out.
- *Inhale* your arms overhead and bring your hands together. Keep the middle of your back touching the wall, even if this means not bringing the palms together.
- *Exhale,* reaching your hands to the right, and breathe into your left ribs. Breathe here easily for five to ten breaths.

- *Inhale*, grounding into your feet, and reach your hands back up so you are vertical again.
- *Exhale*, bringing your hands to the left while keeping your ribs on the wall. Breathe five to ten breaths into your right ribs.
- *Inhale*, grounding deeply, and reach back up to a vertical position.
- *Exhale*, releasing the arms down and rolling the shoulders back and down. Repeat two more times.

6. Widen your feet and explore *Goddess Pose* and then add the *PFCR* as you breathe in the pose. You will exhale and feel your pelvic floor contract when you lower down. Keep breathing naturally while contracting it for a count of ten.

- *Inhale*, releasing your pelvic floor and straightening your legs while rising.
- *Exhale*, lower back into the pose, and engage the pelvic floor contraction for ten breaths.
- *Inhale* as you release the pelvic floor and rise. Repeat in this way for three more cycles.

7. Come to sit in *Staff Pose* on the edge of a folded blanket and breathe five breaths, then move into *Twisted Staff Pose:*

Twisted Staff Pose, *Parivrtta Dandasana*

- *Inhale* while lifting your arms up like a T.
- *Exhale*, twisting to the left while sustaining the rising through the crown of your head. Resist the temptation to lean backward!
- Place your left hand behind you and your right hand on the outside of the left thigh. *Inhale* and lengthen the spine.
- *Exhale*, feeling the core contraction as you twist. Do not jam yourself into this twist more by pressing firming into the

outer thigh. Let your body reveal to you your natural limits for the twist.

- Once in your safe range of motion, release the arms down. Stay in this twist for five breaths.
- *Inhale*, bringing your arms up.
- *Exhale*, untwisting to face forward.
- *Inhale* and lengthen your spine.
- *Exhale* and twist to the right, placing your right hand behind you and your left hand on the outside of the right thigh. Stay in the twist for five breaths.
- Inhale to untwist and return to *Staff Pose*.

8. Come into *Extended Child's Pose* for three to five breaths.

9. Turn onto your back and bring your feet down to the width of your yoga mat for *Windshield Wipers:*

Windshield Wipers

- Lay your arms either alongside you on the mat or out like a T.
- Bend your knees and place your feet as wide as your yoga mat comfortably away from your hips.
- *Inhale* into your belly, back, and ribs.
- *Exhale*, letting your knees fall to the right, and breathe into the ribs.
- *Inhale* your knees to neutral and *exhale*, letting them fall to the left. Again, breathe into the ribs. Let the shoulder blades rise off the mat naturally as your knees move from side to side.
- Continue rocking your knees from right to left on the rhythm of the breath. If desired, turn your head away from the direction of the knees when they fall to either side and bring your head back to the center when your knees face the ceiling. Proceed in this way for one or two minutes.

10. End the practice in *Rest and Relaxation Pose* for at least five minutes.

Note for C-section mothers: If you feel any pulling near or at your incision site, minimize your range of motion with how far you bring your knees toward the floor as you twist from side to side.

Embodied Voice Exploration: Discover the Tonal Current[27]

- Begin by humming on the N consonant. Feel its vibrations on the upper gum ridge.
- Now slowly feel the word "no" and then "yes." The N in "no" brings your awareness to the upper gum ridge.
- Experiment with feeling the vibration of the Y in "yes" at the same spot where you feel the N vibrations. Work slowly but with engaged behavior, meaning you can make believe a friend bought tacky shoes and says, "Aren't these the most elegant shoes you have ever seen?" and you are politely, but tentatively, saying, "YYYes...?"
- Once you feel the rumbling, whirling vibration of the Y, hum on it up and down in your speaking range. Feel how it can move away from the upper gum ridge and onto other surfaces of the mouth.
- After a few vocal slides, let the Y waft down, so you feel it most fully on the upper gum ridge. Sustain the reverse megaphone and relax the tongue to facilitate this movement.
- Breathe. Smile with your eyes. (It helps to do this with your adorable baby. How can you not smile with your eyes when you look at him/her?)
- Now say, "Hi, Cutie," and sustain the Y feeling at the end of "Cutie" in your mid-range, natural speaking voice.
- Add a Y in front of the long E to keep the vibrations moving forward. It will feel like, "Hi, Cutieee—yeee-yeee-yeee-yeee." You are massaging the vocal vibrations forward to the upper

gum ridge and developing a warm, vibrant tone for your speaking voice.

This week, continue playing with the transition from the N consonant to the Y consonant to playfully identify vocal vibrations without needing to have a contact point in the mouth with the tongue.

Meditation: Counting with the Breath

Continue *Counting with the Breath*, but gradually add one or two counts to it so you develop a larger, yet relaxed, breath capacity while stilling the fluctuations of the mind.

Optional: Read about *non-excess* in **Part Four** and journal what you discover about this practice. I encourage you to continue exploring this principle as you move through the program.

Phase Four

For most people, (deep insight into complete absorption of the heart-mind) is preceded by faith, vitality, strong memory, samadhi, then deep insight.
Yoga Sutra 1.20

You have read *Yoga Sutra* 1.20 several times. Each time you have come across it, you have been at a new stage in your path. How do you take it in now? What resonates with you? Stay open to what comes as you meditate on this teaching. Trust your inner-felt teacher.

By now, you are feeling stronger in your core and are more comfortable with the pelvic floor contraction and release exercises. You are feeling musicality in your speaking voice that's enlivening your spirit. Feel how your consonants bring the books you read to your child to life!

The breathing and meditation practices have brought peace and stillness to your inner life. In this phase, we will explore a breathing practice focused on controlling the expansion of the chest and abdomen through which we feel the breath enter and leave the torso. This practice is calming and grounding.

Now that you have established optimal ribs-to-pelvis alignment to strengthen your muscles, you will add squats to the *Movement-Based Practice* and movements that continue your work toward healing diastasis recti.

The *Embodied Voice Practice* will develop your vocal tone, so it feels warm, rich, and pleasant. It brings the vocal vibrations forward to eliminate vocal fry. You will carry over awareness of the musicality of consonants and vocal resonance into feeling children's nursery rhymes. You will notice the tonal color, variety, and natural imagery that comes from within when you feel your voice and speech connect with the rhythm of the stories.

Your *Meditation Practice* includes awareness of your baby as you simultaneously feel your inner landscape.

Community Prompt

Find two or three parents with children of similar ages to yours and set up a playdate at the playground. Even if your baby is small, you can wear him/her in a baby carrier and gently swing with him/her while talking with other parents. Your baby will enjoy seeing kids bigger than him/her play and climb. It's important to have children exposed to a range of ages with varying speaking and movement abilities so they can grow together as a community.

Phase Four, Week One

Breath-Based Practice: Three-Part Breath

This breathing practice brings awareness to the wholeness of breath capacity while also targeting specific respiratory muscles for expansion and release.

Three-Part Breath, *Dirga Pranayama*

- Lie back comfortably with your knees bent and feet on the floor. Feel your spine align on the mat.
- Place one hand on your lower belly and the other on your chest.
- *Inhale,* feeling your breath moving into your belly; *exhale,* release.
- Broaden your awareness of the breath to feeling it in the lower belly, upper belly, and then chest upon inhalation.

- *Exhale* and feel your breath leave your chest, your upper belly, then your lower belly. It's as if your torso were a bucket and the breath fills it from the bottom (lower belly) up (chest) and empties from the top (chest) to the bottom (lower belly).
- Relax and focus on this breath sequence for one to three minutes. This breath allows you to breathe deeply and lower your stress.

Movement-Based Practice: Feel Centered While Getting Strong

1. Review the *Core Foundation* from **Phase One**: *PFCR, Postural Alignment for Healing Diastasis Recti, Hand Corset,* and *Birthday Candle Breath* on an F consonant exhalation. Remember the feeling of the hand corset as you move through your work, so you know how to align your ribs from back to front.
2. Move into *Table Pose* and note the feeling of the hand corset by keeping your ribs aligned, with no lower rib flare.
3. From here, find a slow flow on your breath rhythm, moving from *Cow Pose* (inhale) to *Cat Pose* (exhale) to *Extended Puppy Dog Pose* with a keen awareness of the positioning of the rib alignment (inhale and exhale) back to *Cow Pose* (inhale). Repeat this flow three to five times.
4. Once complete, come onto your belly for *Locust Pose*. Explore this pose two times with awareness of the length of the spine from the middle of the back of the head to the tailbone.
5. Move onto *Table Pose* and through *Bird Dog Pose* for eight repetitions for each side. Move slowly and keep a bodymind feeling of the hand corset as you move.
6. Move into *Modified Side Plank* for eight breaths per side.
7. Come onto your back for *Floor Angels* and notice if you can lower your blanket bolster any due to the strength and length you have gained in your torso over this practice. Move through five *Floor Angel* movements.

8. Come onto your feet for *Mountain Pose* and get grounded through your breath awareness.
   Keep a focus on your ribs-to-pelvis alignment as you add *Eagle Arms* for three to five breaths.

9. Once complete, add *Awkward Chair Pose:*

Awkward Chair Pose, *Utkatasana*

Remember to keep your lower ribs engaged in to keep your spine long and preserve length in your rectus abdominus.

- Begin in *Mountain Pose*, grounding through your feet as you bend your knees, sending your hips down and back as if you're about to sit in a chair.
- Keep your hands on the hips, your breastbone lifted, and the top of your ribs in line with the bottom (no rib flare!). Sustain the pose for three to five breaths.
- Inhale, grounding through your feet to straighten your legs and return to *Mountain Pose.* Repeat two more times. For added adductor (inner thigh) strengthening, hold a yoga block on the thin setting between the thighs as you send your hips down.

10. Come to your back for *Windshield Wipers* for one minute.

11. End your practice with *Rest and Relaxation Pose* for five minutes.

Embodied Voice Exploration: Y Buzz

- Feel the balance of vocal vibration as you move from the N consonant to the Y consonant and sustain your Y consonant on one pitch.
- Feel the word "easy" and notice the ping of vocal vibration on the upper gum ridge (the place you feel the vibration on the

N consonant). Arthur Lessac calls this the "Y buzz," which is a wonderful, therapeutic tool for the voice.

When developing the Y buzz, it is important to sustain the reverse megaphone forward facial orientation and breathe comfortably. Feel the Y consonant with a true long E vowel, smile in the eyes (remember—engaged behavior!), and feel a sense of floating through the crown of your head—just as you felt every time you sat in *Easy Pose* or *kneeling*. If you ever feel a lack of vibration on the upper gum ridge in the Y buzz, check this list and notice what element is missing. Incorporate it and see how these actions all function together.

- Massage the Y buzz with a gentle pulse: "Yeee—yeee-yeee-yeee-yeee."
- Keep breathing naturally; there's no need to push your breath through any of this work.
- Now feel the Y buzz in the following words: **tea leaves, peace, keep, lucky, me, complete, tree, free.**

Once you feel the Y buzz on one pitch, gently slide it up and down a few notes while keeping it on the upper gum ridge. This is called the "tonal current," and it helps develop pitch variety and strengthen the voice. You only need to go up and down a couple of pitches to feel it. You will feel the Y buzz vibrate on the upper gum ridge, the sinus cavity, and in the third eye between the eyebrows.

If sustained for a length of time comfortably with an upright postural alignment, this opening of vibration through the front of the face relaxes your mind and brings your brain into a meditative state. It is a wonderful practice to do while holding your baby.

Meditation: Holding Baby Scan
This phase's meditation can be done whenever you cuddle your baby for comfort. If your child is no longer a baby, you may hold

your child or place your hands on your heart with an image of your child placed there.

- Feel your baby in your arms and focus on your hands. Feel the warmth of your arms and your child in them.
- Feel your hands on your baby as the foreground against the background of your body.
- Feel your heart—front and back—with your awareness of your breath and baby's breath.
- Feel your shoulders and the position of your arms holding your baby but not having to grip. Soften your shoulders where you can.
- Then feel your pelvis connecting you down while supporting the upright alignment of your spine and your child in your arms. Stay here feeling your breath and this loving warmth for as long as possible.

Phase Four, Week Two

Take time to find your intention for this week's practices. Is it different than the last time you investigated it? What keeps you committed to your path? It's your birthright to feel well and be happy. Open yourself toward it and find the work you need to do to sustain it.

Breath-Based Practice: Three-Part Breath with Pleasure Smelling and Pleasure Sighing

Continue exploring the *Three-Part Breath* and add Lessac's teaching of *pleasure smelling* and *pleasure sighing* as your inhalations/ exhalations. Notice if you feel more expansion throughout the trunk when you add a behavioral connection to your breath.

Movement-Based Practice: Adding Strengthening Dynamics

1. Review the *Core Foundation* from Phase One: *PFCR, Postural Alignment for Healing Diastasis Recti, Hand Corset,* and *Birthday Candle Breath* on an F consonant exhalation. Remember the feeling of the hand corset as you move through your work, so you know how to align your ribs from back to front.
2. Move onto *Table Pose* and through *Bird Dog Pose* for eight repetitions for each side. Move slowly and keep a bodymind feeling of the hand corset as you move.
3. Move into *Modified Side Plank* for eight breaths on your left side.
4. Once complete, move through *Clamshells, Inner Thigh Lift,* and *Outer Thigh Lift* for eight repetitions each. Work slowly and focus on your muscle activation and core connections.
5. Repeat *Modified Side Plank* and *Clamshells, Inner Thigh Lift,* and *Outer Thigh Lift* on the right side.
6. Come onto your back for *Floor Angels* and move through the movements of your arms with awareness of your breath and core connections.
7. Come onto your feet for *Mountain Pose* and feel grounded through your breath awareness.
8. Move through three *Half Sun Salutations*.
9. Step the feet wide for *Goddess Pose* for five breaths. Feel *PFCR* on your exhalations.
10. Add *Wide and Parallel Squats (Pulsing)*:

Wide and Parallel Squats (Pulsing)

- Step the feet wide as in *Goddess Pose*. Keep the lower ribs from flaring out by lengthening through the spine. Bring the hands together at the heart and pulse the hips down and up on the breath. If desired, add *PFCR* by inhaling/relaxing the pelvic floor as you pulse the hips down and contracting the pelvic floor as you exhale and pulse up.

- Complete ten pulses before returning to *Mountain Pose.*
- Bring the feet shoulder-width apart and place your hands on your hips or with your palms together at your heart. Pulse your hips down and back for ten breaths. If desired, add PFCR as you did in the wide squat. Sustain the pelvis-to-rib alignment. You may feel the PFCR more strongly in one squat than the other. Note which feels better and perform it daily as part of your pelvic floor regimen.

11. Come to *Staff Pose* and get grounded.

12. Feel the spine get long and release in *Twisted Staff Pose* for five breaths on each side.

13. Lie back for *Supine Crescent Stretch* for five breaths.

14. Rest in *Legs Up the Wall Pose* for three to five minutes.

Embodied Voice Exploration: +Y Buzz

- Feel the Y buzz on both syllables of the word "sleepy." Sustaining the tonal current and reverse megaphone feel in the mouth, feel the word "baby."
- Now go back and forth between the two words "sleepy baby." Notice how the vibrations on the first syllable in "baby" expand a bit but stay focused forward on the upper gum ridge? The vibrations return to the Y buzz on the second syllable.
- Feel it again: "sleepy baby."

The slight expansion of the long A vowel in "baby" is called the +Y buzz. It is also a vowel within the tonal current and will strengthen the voice. It is a diphthong, meaning it has two sounds that come together as one entity. The +Y buzz has the long A followed a shorter long E vowel; it returns to the Y buzz at the end.

- Feel the +Y buzz in "yay, yay, yay, yay." Again, explore with behavior. You can say, "Yay, sleepy baby" or "Yay, baby play with me."
- Massage/pulse the +Y buzz with "Yee, yay." Your mouth will not move much between the Y buzz and the +Y buzz. Sustain the elasticity and vitality of the reverse megaphone while you explore and feel how little you need to do to feel the potency of these two vowels.
- Develop the +Y buzz in the words: **make, cradle, play date, bathe, baby, name, safety, graceful.**

Meditation: Hold Baby Scan

Continue the *Hold Baby Scan* meditation and see if it can carry over to a sense of mindfulness every time you hold your baby. Feel your baby's warmth, size, weight, breathing, and love.

Optional: Read about *non-hoarding* in **Part Four** and journal what you discover about this practice. I encourage you to continue your exploration of this principle as you move through the program.

Phase Four, Week Three

Let each breath that comes in and out be an offering of gratitude. Each inhalation comes from the Divine as thanks for practicing in ways that nurture the gift of you. Each exhalation is a sharing of thanks to the Divine for all you have created and all that surrounds you.

Breath-Based Practice: Continue Three-Part Breath in Various Positions

Continue the *Three-Part Breath* but now explore it in the following positions: lying on your back, sitting in *Easy Pose,* or *kneeling,* and standing in *Mountain Pose.* It may seem more challenging to feel the movement of the three parts of the back/trunk while standing.

If so, return to the position it felt most accessible and notice what parts of your body and mind are free to allow movement. Then work toward carrying that over into standing in *Mountain Pose* to accomplish the same ease of movement with the breath.

Movement-Based Practice: Refined Awareness of Core Connections

This week, you will move with a more refined awareness of core connections from the sequence from **Phase Four, Week One.**

1. Review the *Core Foundation* from Phase One: *PFCR, Postural Alignment for Healing Diastasis Recti, Hand Corset,* and *Birthday Candle Breath* on an F consonant exhalation. Remember the feeling of the hand corset as you move through your work, so you know how to align the ribs from back to front.
2. Move into *Table Pose* and note the feeling of the hand corset by keeping the ribs aligned with no lower rib flare. From here, find a slow flow on your breath rhythm.
3. Move from *Cow Pose* (inhale) to *Cat Pose* (exhale) to *Extended Puppy Dog Pose* with a keen awareness of the positioning of the rib alignment (inhale and exhale), then back to *Cow Pose* (inhale). Repeat this flow five times.
4. Once complete, come onto your belly for *Locust Pose*. Explore this pose two times with a keen awareness of the length of the spine from the middle of the back of the head to the tailbone.
5. Move onto *Table Pose* and then through *Bird Dog Pose* for eight repetitions for each side.
6. Add *PFCR* on your breath, exhaling as you contract the pelvic floor and lift the opposite arm and leg. *Inhale* as you release the movement and relax the pelvic floor contraction. Move slowly and keep a bodymind feeling of the hand corset as you move.

7. Move into *Modified Side Plank* for eight breaths per side.

8. Come onto your feet for *Mountain Pose* and get grounded through your breath awareness.

9. Add *Eagle Arms* for three to five breaths, focusing on your ribs-to-pelvis alignment.

10. Once complete, move into *Awkward Chair Pose* and add arms to the pose this way: Squat as described and lift the arms straight out ahead and up with palms facing each other and in line with the shoulders. Keep the lower ribs in and the back long and strong. You may feel the back activating to support your torso and arms. Sustain the pose for three to five breaths.

11. *Inhale,* grounding through the feet to straighten the legs, lower the arms, and return to *Mountain Pose.* You can also find your way into *Awkward Chair Pose* by beginning in *Tall Mountain Pose* (*Mountain Pose* with the arms elevated over-head) and then sitting the hips back and down. Again, keep the lower ribs in to keep equal in length in the front and back of the torso.

12. Move through eight *Pulsing Squats with PFCR.*

13. Return to *Windshield Wipers* for one minute.

14. End your practice with *Rest and Relaxation Pose* for at least five minutes.

Embodied Voice Exploration: +Y Buzz

This week, you will continue developing consonants and tonal resonance but with an awareness of how you feel these energies while reading a story to your baby. Do you feel the musical rhythm of your consonants while you hum and tap them in words? Do you feel the Y buzz current in your voice while keeping an easy focus of your vocal resonance forward in the mouth? Do you feel this tonal focus easily expand into the +Y buzz whenever it appears (in the long A vowel)?

- Explore the sounds you feel in this commonly told nursery rhyme: "Baa black sheep, have you any wool? Yes, sir, yes, sir, three bags full. One for my master, and one for my dame, and one for the little boy that lives down the lane."
- You will feel:
  - the tap of the K in "black,"
  - the Y buzz in "sheep,"
  - the buzzy V in "have" and the "L" in "wool."
  - The Y buzz will ping the upper gum ridge on "three," and you will feel the rhythm of the "G" and the "S" (felt like a "Z") in "bags" and the hum of the "L" in "full." You will feel:
- the hum of the "N" in "one" and the "S" in "master,"
- the "N" in "and" followed by the tap of the "D,"
- the hum of the "M" in "dame," and
- the tap of the "T" in "little" that doesn't fully spring away, but links to the "L" in "little" (the tip of the tongue doesn't leave the upper gum ridge here).
- This clicking sensation reappears in the link between the "T" and the "L" in "that lives." You will feel:
- the hum of the "V" and the "S" (felt like a "Z") in "lives," and
- the hum of the "N" in "down" and "lane," as well as the +Y buzz in "lane."

There is so much to feel, right? Keeping this connection to what you feel as you speak and read continues your vocal development "off the mat," so you find pleasure in speaking.

Meditation: Hold Baby Scan by Counting with the Breath

Continue the *Hold Baby Scan* while you move through life and see if you can add the *Counting with the Breath Meditation* while you hold the baby at nighttime so you both can relax into a nice sleep at night.

Optional: Read about *cleanliness* in **Part Four** and journal what you discover about this practice. I encourage you to continue your exploration of this principle as you move through the program.

Phase Five

For most people, (deep insight into complete absorption of the heart-mind) is preceded by faith, vitality, strong memory, samadhi, then deep insight.
Yoga Sutra 1.20

Now you are finding more and more *samadhi* (bliss) as you come to stillness. The bliss within radiates outwardly as you take care of your baby, and you feel a difference in how he/she is around you.

Bliss and wellness of spirit are contagious! Let the bodymind lead the way through your practices so you can honor the intelligent teacher within.

In **Phase Five**, you will explore a popular yogic breathing practice that balances the body and mind and brings peace to the spirit. You will continue lengthening and strengthening your core and hips in your *Movement-Based Practice*, so you can find more openness in your mid-back and hips in the movement practice. Your *Embodied Voice Practice* opens into dilute vowels that bring more vocal variety to your vocal life, as well as connecting with the elasticity of the muscles in your jaw, lips, and cheeks. Your *Meditation Practice* dives into the subtle body with a scan of the seven main energy centers called the "*chakras.*"

Community Prompt

Find a park, recreational center, or nature reserve and spend time outdoors in the mid-morning on a pleasant day with your baby. Find parents with their children and engage with them. You can walk a trail together, throw stones in the pond, and observe the animals in this environment. Being in the fresh air and moving around will lift your spirits. You'll find a new place for time away from home, and you can connect with new friends in the outdoors.

Phase Five, Week One

Breath-Based Practice: Alternate Nostril Breathing

Alternate Nostril Breathing calms anxiety, balances both hemispheres of the brain, and prepares the mind and body for meditation.

Alternate Nostril Breathing, *Nadi Shodhana*

- Sit in *Easy Pose, Hero Pose,* or *kneeling* with optimal spinal/rib/pelvis alignment.
- Curl the fingers of the right hand into the palm and release the thumb, ring finger, and pinky. If desired, lay the index and middle fingers on your third eye between your eyebrows.
- Lightly press the thumb on the right nostril and *inhale* through the left nostril. Press the ring finger on the left nostril and *exhale* through the right nostril.
- *Inhale* through the right nostril and press the thumb on the right nostril to *exhale* through the left nostril. Repeat this for one minute, taking care to end the practice by exhaling through the right nostril.
- Release the hand and breathe naturally for one more minute with your eyes closed. Feel the energetic balance between both sides of the body.

Movement-Based Practice: Stabilize and Release the Hips

1. Begin by lying on your back with knees bent for *Semi-Supine Toe Taps.* Add the *Birthday Candle Breath* to the movement

to further engage the transverse abdominus muscle. Work slowly.

2. Move onto *Table Pose* and flow through eight breaths in *Cow Pose* and *Cat Pose* while adding *PFCR*.

3. Once completed, flow through eight repetitions in *Bird Dog Pose*.

4. Come to *Mountain Pose* and flow through five *Half Sun Salutations* with the addition of *Extended Puppy Dog Pose: Inhale—Tall Mountain*, *Exhale*—bent knee standing forward fold with blocks, *Inhale*—extend the spine (flat back), *Exhale*—bend the knees a lot and place hands on the mat and walk feet back until you are in the *Extended Puppy Dog Pose*. Breathe here for three breaths while keeping a keen awareness of the rib-to-pelvis alignment. *Inhale*, walk your feet forward and come to extend the spine (flat back). *Exhale*, standing in a forward fold with the blocks. *Inhale*, bending your knees, grounding through your feet, and rise into *Tall Mountain Pose*. *Exhale*, staying in *Mountain Pose*.

5. Come to *Awkward Chair Pose* for five breaths.

6. Move into *Wide-Leg Pulsing Squats* for five breaths.

7. Go into *Standing Crescent Stretch*, keeping a ribs-to-pelvis alignment.

8. Add *Pyramid Pose:*

Pyramid Pose, *Parsvottanasana*

Keep your lower ribs engaged in, shortening your stride a bit more than what you would pre-pregnancy.

- Begin in *Mountain Pose*.
- Step your left foot back while keeping your hip bones facing forward and your pelvis in line with the spine.
- Soften your right knee, place your hands on your hips, and bend forward from the hip crease while lengthening the

breastbone. Only move as far forward as you feel a slight stretch in the outer hips—not the spine—and keep a keen connection to the back of the core, supporting the weight of your torso as you lean forward. Keep a bend in your front knee to ease into the pose.

- Breathe here for five breaths. *Inhale*, grounding through the right foot to raise the torso, and step the left foot forward to return to *Mountain Pose*.
- Repeat for the other side.

9. Come into *Staff Pose*, then feel your breath lengthening your spine in *Twisted Staff Pose* for five breaths on the left and five on the right.

10. Add *#4 Legs Pose:*

#4 Legs Pose

- Sit on the edge of a firm folded blanket and extend your legs as in *Staff Pose*.
- Bend your right knee and cross the outside of your right shin on top of your left thigh as if making the number "4" with your legs.
- Sit tall and breathe into the outer hips. Micro-fold from the hip crease to further lengthen the muscles surrounding the outer hips. It doesn't take much to feel the release. Breathe here for five breaths.

11. Rest in *Windshield Wipers* for two to three minutes.

12. Come into *Rest and Relaxation Pose* for five minutes.

Embodied Voice Exploration: Attune with the Mouth's Inner Space

We have opportunities in our speech in which we don't feel any vocal resonance or have any tactile sensations on the bony surfaces of the mouth. Many vowels are known as "dilute," which means they aren't concentrated with vocal vibration like the tonal vowels. Yet just because they are not rich with sensation doesn't mean you cannot feel them nor feel connected to the beauty of your voice through them. For example, feel the magnificence in Anton Chekhov's line from *The Seagull*: "You have found your path; you know which way you are going. But I'm still whirled about in a maze of dreams and images, not knowing what it is all about and who wants it."

There's a lovely lightness in many of the vowels that open a speaker to the vulnerability and heartbreak the character communicates. Similarly, we can open ourselves more fully to the inherent essence of what we speak when we lean into the softer side of our expressive selves. We can explore that arena through the dilute vowels. When we experience the dilute vowels with the tone and richness of consonants and tonal vowels, we come into a myriad of sensations as we speak that we emote our expressive and authentic selves with conviction, truth, and freedom.

We often shy away from expressing our truest desires by barely opening our mouths to speak. We, in a sense, swallow our voices and only speak when we need to. Conversely, we might shout through this swallowed voice forcefully and suffer a sore throat much of the time.

Consider this a signal to free your voice and tap into an expression that communicates your need while also liberating you to express your wants.

- Start by opening your mouth as large as possible *without* unhinging your jaw. You will feel it the same way you open it when your doctor asks to look at the back of your throat.
- Continue feeling the reverse megaphone and notice how large the lip opening can become while feeling the lift in the back of the throat and the length of the sides of the cheeks.

- Now move from that large lip opening to the smallest circle you can *comfortably* make without tension. You can blow a small stream of air through this circle.
- Then move from the large lip opening to the small circle and notice the muscular action of the lips and cheeks along the way. Do this slowly but without holding or tensing anything as you move. Repeat it with voice and without (a bare whisper).

Your lips are moving through many dilute vowels whether your voice makes them fully or not. Your work now is to discover the size and shape of the lip opening that creates a particular sound. In this manner, you speak a vowel sound without needing to hear it or feel it resonate in the mouth, but by feeling the muscular action of the lips and cheeks that creates it.

Feel the elasticity of the cheeks and lips as you say "Woo-Woe-War-Wah-Wow-Why." Play with this phrase with vocal tone and as a barely audible whisper.

Meditation: Chakra Scan

The *chakras* are powerful energy centers that align the spine in seven locations. You can determine balances and imbalances in the subtle body with an attunement with the *chakras*. Follow my cues to feel where they are and breathe naturally into each one.

- Notice the breath moving into the abdomen and the pelvis. Bring awareness to the pelvic floor and feel its movement. Attune with the root *chakra* at the pelvic floor. Imagine its swirling action moving from left to right in a subtle whirlpool effect.
- Stay there for several breaths. Then bring awareness to the lower belly between the hip bones to the sacral *chakra*. You may feel it swirling from left to right.

- After several breaths, bring awareness to the area at the upper belly between the lower rib cage to the solar plexus *chakra*. Breathe here for several breaths.
- Bring your awareness to the heart *chakra* in the center of the chest. Breathe here for several breaths while noticing your child in this space.
- Then bring awareness to the throat *chakra*. Notice if you have things left unsaid congesting this area.
- Then bring awareness to the area between the eyebrows for the third eye *chakra*. Notice any intuition or insights that come to you when you breathe into this space.
- Then bring awareness to the crown of the head for the crown *chakra*. It will swirl from left to right horizontally to your head, like how the root *chakra* moved at the pelvic floor. The crown *chakra* connects you to the universe and God.
- After scanning each *chakra* individually, feel all seven as a collective while running up the length of the spine. Breathe easily.

Phase Five, Week Two

As you sit in meditation this week, feeling your breath and scanning the energy centers along the spine, seek with curiosity where absolute beauty and grace lie within. Where do you feel them most? Notice how you can be so open in these areas that beauty and grace reveal themselves. Let the bodymind teach the other parts of you how to open themselves to beauty and grace such that the whole of you shines from the inside out.

Breath-Based Practice: Alternate Nostril Breathing

Continue *Alternate Nostril Breathing* and add *Even Ratio Breathing* to balance the rhythm of your breath cycle.

Movement-Based Practice: Diving More Deeply Within for Strength and Support

1. Begin by lying on your back with knees bent for *Semi-Supine Toe Taps*. Add the *Birthday Candle Breath* to the movement to further engage the transverse abdominus muscle. Work slowly.
2. Move onto *Table Pose* and flow through eight breaths in *Cow Pose* and *Cat Pose* while adding *PFCR*.
3. Once completed, flow through eight repetitions in *Bird Dog Pose*.
4. Come to *Mountain Pose* and flow through five *Half Sun Salutations* with the addition of *Extended Puppy Dog Pose*.
5. Feel *Pyramid Pose* for eight breaths on each side with a focus on core activation throughout the pose, particularly in the back of the body.
6. Add *Extended Side Angle Pose:*

Extended Side Angle Pose, *Utthita Parsvakonasana*
Keep your lower ribs engaged in and shorten your stride by 30% of what you would do pre-pregnancy.

- Begin in *Mountain Pose* at the center of the mat, facing the long side of the mat. Step your feet wide, then shorten your stride by about 30% to preserve the ligament at the center of your pubic bone.
- Pivot on the heel of your right foot so your toes face the short side of the mat.
- Pivot on the left heel to bring your toes in about 30 degrees.
- Bend your right knee and place your right forearm on your right thigh. Keep your lower ribs engaged inward to preserve length in the front and back of your torso.

- *Inhale,* extending your left arm on the diagonal so it hovers just ahead of your left ear with the palm facing down. Sustain the pose for five breaths.
- Ground through your right foot to lift the torso to a vertical position while returning your left arm to its original position.
- Straighten your right leg and change sides by pivoting your feet appropriately, bending your left knee and placing your left forearm on your thigh.
- Extend your right arm up and breathe five breaths. Ground through your feet as you exit the pose and return to *Mountain Pose* by walking your feet forward a few inches at a time.

7. Come to sit in *Staff Pose* to feel grounded.
8. Explore *Seated Wide-Legged Forward Fold Pose:*

Seated Wide-Legged Forward Fold Pose, *Upavistha Konasana*

- Sit on a firm folded blanket and bring your legs wide with your feet active as if you are standing on them.
- Now shorten your stride by about 30% to preserve the ligament at the center of your pubic bone.
- Place your hands either inside your inner thighs on a yoga block or place them outside of your hips.
- Lengthen your spine and breathe for three breaths.
- *Inhale* your arms forward and up to shoulder height.
- *Exhale,* reaching your torso forward while keeping a micro-bend in the knees. Only go as far forward as you can while keeping length in your spine. Don't round it or thrust out your lower ribs. Feel the back of the core supporting you.
- Once you find an appropriate fold, place your hands down and breathe five breaths.
- *Inhale,* walking your hands toward you to safely come out of the pose.

- Bend your knees, bring your legs together, and breathe three breaths in *Staff Pose*.

9. Feel *#4 Legs Pose* for eight breaths on each side, keeping your spine long.

10. Add *Marichi's Pose C:*

Marichi's Pose C, *Marichyasana* C

Keep this pose gentle and focus on lengthening your spine.

- Begin in *Staff Pose.* Keep your left leg extended and in line with your hip joint.
- Bend your right leg and place your right foot a couple of inches from your left inner thigh. Sit tall—if your lower back rounds because you placed your foot toward the pelvis, either move the foot farther away or sit on an additional firm blanket. Keep your lower back long and feel tall through the crown of the head.
- *Inhale,* raising your left arm to shoulder height.
- *Exhale,* twisting to the right, and then wrap your left arm *around* your bent leg as if you are hugging yourself. Do *not* bring your elbow to the outside of your thigh, as this put too much strain on the ligaments of your pelvis.
- Place your right hand behind you. Keep sitting tall—*inhale* to lengthen the spine; *exhale* to engage in the twist. Breathe five breaths.
- *Inhale,* releasing your left arm and untwist; *exhale,* returning to *Staff Pose.*
- Bend your left knee and place your left foot on the floor where it feels appropriate for your lower back.
- Repeat this pose on the other side.

11. Complete your practice with one to two minutes of *Windshield Wipers* before coming into *Rest and Relaxation Pose* for five minutes.

Note for C-section mothers: Minimize your range of motion in your mid-to-low back as you twist if you feel any pulling near or at your incision site. You can keep the twist in your upper back and progress to more fully incorporating your mid back as you heal and get stronger.

Embodied Voice Exploration: Introducing the Dilute Vowels

Lessac identifies 11 dilute vowels in American English, all with unique lip opening sizes and shapes. [Note: there are many more vowel sounds possible with voice and speech, including many beautiful sounds made in languages and dialects outside of American English.] Here, we will develop five of them.[28] His use of sizes and shapes are guidelines for how you feel space and movement in the mouth as you speak.

The most important aspect of feeling dilute vowels is attuning with the space inside the mouth that the reverse megaphone creates. The lengthening of the cheek muscles forward and the accommodating shape and size of the lips will create the dilute vowel such that you feel connected to the vowel's dynamic. When you explore the accompanying word lists with each vowel, allow yourself to feel your natural dialect so long as you feel space and energy in the mouth, cheeks, and lips.

The first is a familiar sound. It's where you started by opening your mouth as if at the doctor's office. Feel this again and notice the oval shape your lips make. Again, please don't unhinge the jaw but yawn into it by engaging the reverse megaphone. This is AH, as in "a ha!"

Lessac assigns numbers to these vowels to resist any temptation to overthink their creation and calls this one #5 (The number assignments are simply a guide for categorizing the different shapes we make.) We naturally feel and say this vowel when inspired: "Ah, yes!" It's an organic impulse to open our mouths when our creativity is stirred, and our spirits inspired.

Feel the oval lip opening feed the sound of the following words (please move your lips to communicate the sound, but yawn into the oval shape of the AH vowel when it appears): **father, card, large, heart, march, arms, darling, park.**

The next sound is also familiar—it's the smallest circular lip opening we can comfortably make. Feel the voice in this shape, and it's "oo." We naturally feel and say this when we are intrigued by something and say "ooo, really?" Lessac calls this the #1 since it comes from a very small circular opening of the lips. We feel the small circle feeding the sound in the following words: **moon, two, shoe, mood, do, you, beautiful, coo.**

The next sound also comes from a circular lip opening. We feel a slightly larger circle with the lips and return to the smallest circle from before. The vowel sound that occurs here—"O" as in "Oh!"—is called a diphthong because it is two different sounds that blend to make one unique sound. Thus, our lips move from the slightly larger circle to the smallest circle to create the "Oh." Lessac calls this the #21 since it goes from a slightly larger circle (the #2) to the #1; thus, it is the #21. [This lip movement is more common in American English. If you do not speak American English, you will feel something slightly different. Enjoy your version of this vowel!] We open into this sound with these words: **old, don't, moment, over, low, cold, both, phone.**

The next sound we will develop is by returning to the #5, AH. Again, yawn into this opening without forcing the jaw. The opening will yield itself the more we feel a yawn-like sensation over time. For now, we return to the familiar opening of the mouth to say "AH" at the doctor and then move the lips to the #1. Feel this several times and notice the sound that comes. This "OW" vowel is called the #51 since it moves from the #5 to the #1 vowel. We explore this vowel through the reverse megaphone shape of the mouth to resist any temptation to pull back the corners of the lips, compromising the integrity of the forward-moving action of the vocal stream. We feel the #51 in these words: **loud, cow, aloud, our, house, pout, proud, devour.**

The last dilute vowel we will develop also begins by feeling the #5. We flatten the blade of the tongue a bit and notice how the corners of the mouth soften a little. We feel the voice in this shape and move toward the Y buzz. We notice the movement happening here not just with the lips and cheeks but also the voice as it becomes the "I" sound. This is called the #6y vowel, and it is the most vulnerable of the vowels because we open the mouth fully to feel it at its best. So, yes, our hearts can shine through our voices by saying "I." We feel the "I" in the phrase "I love you" and notice how the heart softens when we feel the "I" in the phrase. The touch of tonal resonance at the end of "I" feels grounding. We can say "I" and feel vulnerable and grounded at once. There's nothing better! Now feel the #6y in these words: **like, eye, kind, shy, aisle, cry, mine, confide.**

Meditation: Chakra Scan

Continue the *Chakra Scan Meditation* and spend time on areas that feel weak or imbalanced. Breathe into them. Inquire from where the imbalance comes. Don't get lost in the story; honor the sensation, allow your body and mind to release, and adapt to what the *chakras* reveal. This meditation could take up to ten minutes and lead you into a longer investigation of yourself in meditation.

Optional: Read about *contentment* in **Part Four** and journal what you discover about this practice. I encourage you to continue your exploration of this principle as you move through the program.

Phase Five, Week Three

Let the vitality you feel for your practice carry over into all the other work you do to take care of yourself, your baby, your family, and your household. These elements of your life work together to create the oneness within which you live. If you feel fabulous and integrated as you move through your *Embodied Voice Practice*, let that energy inspire you as you tidy up the house or share the day's news with your partner or a friend.

Breath-Based Practice: Alternate Nostril Breathing

Continue *Alternate Nostril Breathing* but this time, move through the feeling without using your hands. Close your eyes and hone your awareness on your left nostril as you breathe in, then shift to the right nostril as you breathe out. Allow your hands to rest comfortably on your lap. Continue in this way for five breath cycles. Note that you can enjoy this breathing practice while holding your baby and in a still, quiet moment.

Movement-Based Practice: Exploring New Dynamics

1. Begin in *Staff Pose* breathing with the *Birthday Candle Breath*. Feel the *Hand Corset* and engage the muscles in the body's midline. Work slowly. Move onto *Table Pose* and flow through eight breaths in *Cow Pose* and *Cat Pose* while adding *PFCR*.
2. Once completed, flow through eight repetitions in *Bird Dog Pose*.
3. Come to *Mountain Pose* for five breaths, then feel *Standing Crescent Stretch* for five breaths on each side.
4. Step back into *Pyramid Pose* for eight breaths on each side with a focus on core activation throughout the pose, particularly in the back of the body, as well as feeling long in the waist. Remember that "activation" means a balanced effort between engagement and release of the muscles with the breath.
5. Step into *Goddess Pose* for eight breaths and focus on strength and stability in the hips.
6. Move into *Extended Side Angle Pose* for eight breaths per side with a focus on strength in the hips, resisting low rib flare, and keeping length on both sides of the waist. You may

not bend as much with these components in place, which is perfectly fine.

7. Move into *Staff Pose*.

8. Add *Cow Face Pose:*

Cow Face Pose, *Gomukhasana*

- Sit on the edge of a firm folded blanket and start in the *#4 Legs Pose* with your right leg bent.
- Move toward stacking your right knee on top of your left knee and breathe. If appropriate for your knees and hips and you have no discomfort, lean back on your hands, and bend your left knee so your foot is near your pelvis. This is the base for *Cow Face Pose*. (Here, you can sit and nurse, give your baby a bottle, or roll your shoulders back.)
- Raise your arms like a T and hold a yoga strap in your left hand.
- Reach your left hand up and bend your left elbow while letting the strap dangle behind you.
- Rotate your right shoulder inward so your right palm faces the wall behind you, then bend your elbow and grab the strap.
- Inch your right hand close to your left. Keep your lower ribs engaged in and feel length in your spine. Breathe five breaths here. **If you feel any tension or force in the shoulders in this pose, release the strap and do Shoulder Rolls instead.**
- Release the strap, lean back on your hands, and uncross your legs.
- Return to *Staff Pose* for five breaths before repeating *Cow Face Pose* for the other side. The side of the body that's the top leg is opposite to the arm on top (right leg, left arm; left leg, right arm).

9. From *Cow Face Pose*, come into *Extended Child's Pose* for three breaths to release the hips.

10. Add *Bridge Pose:*

Bridge Pose, *Setu Bandha Sarvangasana*

- Engage your lower ribs toward the spine to preserve the tone of the muscles of the rectus abdominus. This pose will lengthen the transverse abdominus and strengthen the hips and pelvic floor, even if you keep back-bending to a minimum and your hips lower.
- Lie on the floor with your knees bent and feet hip distance apart. Explore two or three pelvic tilts to ensure the abdomen and hips are relaxed and aligned.
- Lay your hands alongside the body with palms facing down.
- *Inhale,* lengthening your spine.
- *Exhale,* engaging through the feet, shoulder blades, and back of the head to lift your hips about six inches. Keep your lower ribs engaged in toward the spine. Breathe here for five breaths.
- Slowly roll back down, starting with the upper back, middle back, lower back, then the pelvis. Repeat once more for five breaths.

11. Release with the *Extended Child's Pose* for three breaths.

12. Come onto your back for *Rest and Relaxation Pose* for at least five minutes.

Embodied Voice Exploration: Dilute Vowels and Tonal Sentences

Now that we have developed the consonants, tonal vowels, and dilute vowels, it's time to feel the variety in communication. There is a truly sparkling interchange of rhythm and tonal color in the mouth when we speak with awareness. We speak in the tonal current in our daily life. We always want a warm speaking voice that sustains a therapeutic quality for our vocal folds every time we hum on the Y buzz. From this vocal stream, we can feel the taps and hums of the consonants and open into the dilute vowels while returning to the tonal current for the completion of the sound. In this way, we are interested in our voice and speech. We feel like we are singing when we are speaking (a feeling Arthur Lessac jubilantly prompted his students to explore), and we freely express ourselves in ways that energize our spirits.

I suggest you experiment with the dance of the three vocal dynamics whenever you read to your baby or speak daily. Board books are wonderful resources for exploring different ways to express a story simply by focusing your awareness on consonants, tonal vowels, and dilute vowels. You can read one story three times and have three different experiences!

Feel the following sentences to play with the fun musicality of voice and speech:

- Hum on consonants that end syllables and words but not on those that begin words, so you don't impede a flow to the rhythm.
- Tap fully on consonants that similarly end syllables or words and don't have a voiced vowel following (the silent "e" doesn't count—it's silent!).
- Feel the Y buzz as it occurs in words. You will feel the ping of vibration on your upper gum ridge. Realize that some Y buzz opportunities are naturally shorter than others (the difference between "tea leaves" and Y buzz that ends "simply").

In the four sentences below, the vowels developed are in bold, but you will discover movement on the other vowels, too:

1. **My** baby loves **to** play and sleep all **day**.
2. Please **eat** the beans that **we** grew from **our** garden.

3. My father is shy but loves to dance to old time music.
4. Whenever I think of my life, I could cry because I am so happy.

Now feel the dynamics in these sentences that may express frustration. I include these because it is important to feel authentic and connected to your voice even when you do not feel well in the circumstances such as these:

- Please, darling, I need to rest for five minutes. I am so tired.
- My partner came into the house too loudly and woke the baby.
- The baby needs more diapers, and I don't have a car to go buy some.
- It took me eighteen minutes to change the baby's clothes because the phone kept ringing. Now I am late.

Meditation: Chakra Scan

This week, you will continue the *Chakra Scan Meditation* and bring equal awareness to what you feel energetically in the front and back of the body. You tend to scan the *chakras* scanning the *front* line of your body, but what do you discover along the *back* line? You may realize back pain is attributed to a *chakra* that you can release simply through your awareness and breathing practices.

Optional: Read about *discipline* in **Part Four** and journal what you discover about this practice. I encourage you to continue your exploration of this principle as you move through the program.

Phase Six

For most people, (deep insight into complete absorption of the heart-mind) is preceded by faith, vitality, strong memory, samadhi, then deep insight. Intense momentum of practice and faith accelerates them toward samadhi.
Yoga Sutras 1.20-1.21

Notice that the second part of the *Yoga Sutras* lesson from the Introduction has become part of the opening reminder for **Phase Six**. By now, you have found the sequential elements of *Yoga Sutra* 1.20 as true to life. Now notice the momentum these components have as they synergize with one another. It's a wonderful energy that motivates and inspires you on your path.

In this phase, we explore a breathing practice that connects the movement of the breath with a directed focus on the mind throughout the body. We focus the movement practice on refining all movements done thus far and integrating the core connections with awareness of how the movements of the core work with that of the breath. We begin to add spinal flexion to movements because we have developed sufficient strength in the core to support the forward movement of the spine.

In addition, our work on correcting diastasis recti ought to have brought some closure to the spacing between the two abdominal sheaths to explore small forward folds safely. The *Embodied Voice Practice* brings the musicality of the speaking voice into the singing voice as we sing to our little ones and explore popular yogic chants. We focus on feeling the energy of our consonants, vocal tone, and dilute vowels as they synergize in different forms of expression.

Our *Meditation Practice* explores subtler attention inward on two popular *mantras.* We can similarly carry over singing into the yoga practice of chanting *mantras.*

A *mantra* is a word or phrase repeated in meditation to align with its content while feeling the vibration of the word or phrase as a point of meditative focus. *Mantras* focus the mind on liberating your spirit through how you feel the chant, even if you imagine the chant in your mind's eye.

Community Prompt

Invite to your home two or three of the parents you have enjoyed meeting in previous phases for a potluck lunch. It doesn't need to be anything fancy—one person provides the veggies, one brings fruit, and you can make sandwiches or lentils and rice. Notice how fun it can be to share a meal with friends and let the time be leisurely. While you are connecting with your friends, the babies can interact on a play mat together. Don't stress about having a clean home for this gathering. They will understand if there are small messes here and there!

Phase Six, Week One

Breath-Based Practice: River Breath

This week, you will use a meditative breath called *River Breath.*

- Begin by lying comfortably on your back with your knees bent or your legs straight. You may like to place a rolled blanket under your knees to act as a bolster. You may also like to add a folded blanket at the base of your shoulder blades to open the chest. If this strains your neck, add a folded blanket or a book under your head as a pillow.
- Breathe in and feel your breath moving up your nose and sinus cavity, past the third eye, the crown of the head, and

back down the third eye at the back of the head, the back of your throat, the back of your heart, the back of your upper belly (solar plexus), the back of your lower belly (sacral *chakra*), the back of your perineum (root), and moving again through each *chakra* up the front of your body until it leaves your nose past the throat *chakra*. You will feel the flow of the breath as even and smooth.

Movement-Based Practice: Exploring Forward Folds

1. Begin by reviewing the *Core Foundations: PFCR* exercises while lying on your back with your knees bent, sitting upright, and finding *Optimal Postural Alignment* of the pelvis, ribs, head, *Hand Corset,* and *Birthday Candle Breath,* ending with the exhalation on the S consonant.
2. Move into *Table Pose* and flow from *Cow Pose* to *Cat Pose* on the rhythm of your breath while also engaging PFCR. Feel ten of these flows as you inhale in *Cow Pose* (relax the pelvic floor) and exhale in *Cat Pose* (contract the pelvic floor).
3. Move into *Bird Dog Pose* and add *spinal flexion* on the *exhalation.* Inhale, lengthening by putting out your opposing arm and leg. *Exhale,* rounding your spine while engaging your knee and elbow toward each other; *inhale,* extend them back out. *Exhale,* placing your knee and elbow down into *Table Pose.* Do five of these per side. Keep an awareness of rib-to-pelvis alignment.
4. Come to *Easy Pose* on a folded blanket and move through *Six Directions for the Spine.*
5. Come to standing and flow through five *Half Sun Salutations* with the addition of *Extended Puppy Dog Pose.*
6. Once completed, step back into *Pyramid Pose* for eight breaths per side.
7. Come to *Staff Pose* on a folded blanket to support the pelvis.

8. Add *Seated Forward Fold Pose:*

Seated Forward Fold Pose, *Paschimottanasana*

Keep your lower ribs engaged in; keep a bend in the knees to focus your movement on bringing the chest and thighs toward each other and not by rounding the back.

- Bend your knees and place a yoga strap on the balls of your feet, holding the strap like the reins of a horse.
- *Inhale,* lengthening your spine tall, and bring your arms up in front to shoulder height.
- *Exhale,* fold at the hip crease, and bring your chest toward your thighs. Bend your knees as much as you need to for this to happen. Keep the lower ribs engaged in.
- Once you fold as far forward as you comfortably can, place your arms down and hold onto the outside of your legs (or feet) where appropriate. Keep your spine long and your breastbone lengthening. Don't round your back. Breathe here for five breaths.
- *Inhale* to come up and roll the shoulders back.

9. Sit tall and breathe five breaths per side in *Marichi's Pose C* starting with your twist to the right side (right leg bent). Keep your arm around the shin of the bent leg.

10. Lie back and feel five breaths in *Bridge Pose*. Repeat *Bridge Pose* two more times.

11. Rest in *Extended Child's Pose* for three breaths.

12. Come into *Rest and Relaxation Pose* for at least five minutes.

Embodied Vocal Exploration: Singing to the Baby

It's one thing to feel like you are singing while speaking; it's another to sing in daily life. Singing lightens the spirit, opens the voice, relaxes and energizes you in body, mind, and spirit. Singing helps your baby discover musicality, recognize different vocal pitches, and understand reciprocal communication. When your baby coos at you in a particular note or cadence, you can sing it back. The vocal mirroring will affirm his/her identity, attach your baby securely to you, and create a fun game that can last for years! If your child is no longer a baby, you can still enjoy this exploration as an opportunity to connect with yourself.

I would make songs about my daughter and sing them in the car when I couldn't be in the backseat with her. I wanted her to know I was connected with her. Five years later, her face still lights up when I sing these songs.

Try this game:

- Look at your baby and sing, "I love you, (name)." Now sing this phrase with your baby's name in different dynamics. You can focus on the humming through the consonants one way, humming through any Y buzz or +Y buzz words another way, or open your mouth and heart fully on the dilute vowels in another way.
- Sing the phrase going up and down in pitch. See how your baby responds to your voice.
- Let your awareness circle back to yourself and ask:
- How do you feel while you sing in a way in which you sense the vibrations of your voice?
- Do you connect with the content of what you say?
- Can you see the wonder and beauty of your baby as you sing it? When this happens, it's quite a marvelous event!

Meditation: Soham

This week, we meditate on the *mantra* "Soham," which means "I Am That." It is pronounced "So" "Hum." You will not actively chant but say/hear it in your third eye *chakra* with each breath. *Inhale,* feel grounded; *exhale,* feel the *mantra.* Continue in this way for five minutes.

Optional: Read about *self-study* in **Part Four** and journal what you discover about this practice. I encourage you to continue your exploration of this principle as you move through the program.

Phase Six, Week Two

Intense momentum of practice and faith accelerates them toward samadhi.
Yoga Sutra 1.21

Tap into the momentum of practice and faith as you add more elements to the practices this week. Trust that you know all that has come before and open yourself to the newness of what's to come.

Breath-Based Practice: River Breath

Continue exploring *River Breath* as a meditative and centering practice. Try this practice at bedtime.

Movement-Based Practice: From Strength Comes Flexibility

1. Begin by reviewing the *Core Foundations*: *PFCR* exercises while lying on your back with your knees bent, sitting upright, and finding *Optimal Postural Alignment* of pelvis, ribs, and head, *Hand Corset*, and *Birthday Candle Breath*, ending with the exhalation on the S consonant.
2. Move into *Table Pose* and flow from *Cow Pose* to *Cat Pose* on the rhythm of your breath while also engaging *PFCR*. Feel ten of these flows as you inhale in *Cow Pose* (relax the pelvic floor) and exhale in *Cat Pose* (contract the pelvic floor).
3. Move into *Bird Dog Pose* and add *spinal flexion* on the exhalation.
4. Come onto your belly for a flow in *Locust Pose*.

   • Start in *Locust Pose* and raise your chest and legs on the exhale.

- *Inhale*, coming down, and place your hands on either side of the chest. *Exhale*, pressing up into *Table Pose*.
- *Inhale*, lengthening the spine; *exhale* and bring the hips back into *Extended Child's Pose*.
- *Inhale*, lengthening the spine; *exhale* and bring the hips back into *Extended Puppy Dog Pose*.
- *Inhale*, lengthening the spine; *exhale* and come back into *Table Pose*.
- *Inhale*, lengthening the spine; *exhale* and return to *Locust Pose*. Repeat this flow two more times.

5. Come to stand and feel five breaths in *Awkward Chair Pose*.

6. Feel five breaths in *Pulsing Squats* with *PFCR*.

7. Come to the floor into *Cow Face Pose* and add a *Side Bend:* When your left arm is the upper arm, slowly side bend to the right and breathe into the side ribs. *Inhale* to come up and repeat when then right arm becomes the upper arm and bend to the left. Feel five breaths per side.

8. Bring your legs long into *Staff Pose* on a folded blanket and slowly fold forward using a strap for *Seated Forward Fold*.

9. Add *Seated Wide-Legged Forward Fold Pose:*

Seated Wide-Legged Forward Fold Pose (with Twist), *Parivrtta Upavistha Konasana*

- Bring your legs wide with your feet active as if you are standing on them. Shorten your stride by about 30% to preserve the ligament at the center of the public bone.
- Place your hands in front of you, lengthen your spine on an inhalation, and walk your hands forward as you exhale, taking care to hinge at the hip crease. Only go as far forward as you can while keeping length in your spine. Don't round it or thrust out your lower ribs.

- Once you find an appropriate fold, place your hands down and breathe five breaths.
- *Inhale*, then walk your hands toward you to safely come out of the pose.
- Next, bend your right knee and loop a strap at the ball of your foot. Extend your leg, lengthen your spine, and fold over your right leg. Breathe here for three breaths.
- *Inhale* as you rise. Place the strap at the ball of your left foot.
- *Inhale*, lengthening the spine.
- *Exhale*, folding forward over the left leg. Breathe here for three breaths.
- *Inhale*, bend your knees, slowly come up, and bring your legs together. Breathe three breaths in *Staff Pose*.

10. Add *Cobbler's Pose:*

Cobbler's Pose, *Baddha Konasana*

- Sit on the edge of a firm folded blanket and bring the soles of your feet together, drawn toward the pelvis. Bring your feet a little farther away than what you feel you can do to preserve the ligament at the center of the pubic bone. If there is any strain in the knees, hips, or lower back, place yoga blocks under your knees or thighs.
- Hold your feet together and sit tall. Lengthen your spine and keep your lower ribs engaged inwardly. Breathe here for five to ten breaths. This is a wonderful pose for including pelvic floor contraction and release exercises.
- *Inhale,* releasing the pelvic floor; exhale, engaging the pelvic floor in and up. Feel the inward engagement of the lower belly as you contract the pelvic floor.
- *Inhale*, release everything and repeat. At the end of five to ten breaths, let the hands help the knees come together and extend your legs out in *Staff Pose* for three breaths.

11. End your practice with five minutes of *Rest and Relaxation Pose*.

Embodied Vocal Exploration: Singing Favorite Children's Songs

You can extend your vocal awareness to common children's songs such as "Itsy Bitsy Spider," "Twinkle Little Star," and "Baa Black Sheep." Feel each for the rhythm of their consonants and the feeling of the vowels. If you attune to these musical sensations, you can better connect with the song's story and make it even more fun for you to sing and your baby to enjoy.

You find the words to these songs here so you can see how to mark them for awareness of each. Lessac teaches underlining tapped consonants that do not precede a voiced vowel once and double underlining hummable consonants that do not precede a voiced vowel. You would mark above Y buzz vowels with a dot and +Y buzz vowels with a plus sign. You would place an arc above the dilute vowels.

> The itsy, bitsy spider walked up the waterspout
> Down came the rain and washed the spider out
> Up came the sun and dried up all the rain
> And the itsy-bitsy spider walked up the spout again.

> Twinkle, twinkle little star
> How I wonder what you are
> Up above the world so high
> Like a diamond in the sky
> Twinkle, twinkle little star
> How I wonder what you are!

> Baa, baa black sheep have you any wool?
> Yes, sir, yes, sir three bags full
> One for my master, one for my dame
> And one for the little boy who lives on my lane.

Meditation: Hamsa

Now meditate on the *mantra* "Hamsa" (pronounced "hum" "suh") and notice if it grounds you differently than the *mantra* "Soham."

Inhale, think "Ham;" *exhale*, think "Sa." Spend time with "Hamsa" this week and determine which *mantra* you prefer for connecting with your inner light.

Phase Six, Week Three

For most people, (deep insight into complete absorption of the heart-mind) is preceded by faith, vitality, strong memory, samadhi, then deep insight. Intense momentum of practice and faith accelerates them toward samadhi.
Yoga Sutras 1.20-1.21

This is the week you find ownership of the practices if you haven't done so already. Trust in your inherent knowledge, faith, and deep-felt intelligence to what sustains and nourishes your body, mind, voice, spirit, and soul in your *Movement-Based Practice*. Spend time with this in your *Breath-Based Practice* and *Meditation Practice*. Inquire what elements of your life also nurture you and put your energy into these avenues as well. All the elements of life balance each other and we benefit from the stability and vitality they bring us.

Breath-Based Practice: Your Favorite Practice!

This week, enjoy whichever breath-based practice from the program that most grounded and centered you for your move-ment-based practice and activities for the rest of the day. Explore whether you can enjoy this practice in the morning when you arise or when you have a few minutes of quiet during the day and again before bedtime.

Movement-Based Practice: Finding Length in Strength

This week, we will repeat the sequence from **Phase Six, Week Two** with a few additions. Please keep in mind the synchronization of the breath and the deep core muscles.

1. Begin your work reviewing the Core Foundations: *Pelvic Floor Contraction and Relaxation* (PFCR) exercises while lying on your back with your knees bent, sitting upright, and finding an *optimal postural alignment* of the pelvis, ribs, and head, *Hand Corset,* and *Birthday Candle Breath* ending with the exhalation on the S consonant.

2. Move into *Table Pose* and flow from *Cow Pose* to *Cat Pose* on the rhythm of your breath while also engaging *PFCR*. Feel ten of these flows as you inhale in *Cow Pose* (relax the pelvic floor) and exhale in *Cat Pose* (contract the pelvic floor).

3. Move into *Bird Dog Pose* and add *spinal flexion* on the exhalation.

4. Come onto your belly for the flow, starting and ending with *Locust Pose.* Complete four repetitions.

5. Come onto your left side for *Modified Side Plank* for eight breaths.

6. Explore the series of *Clamshells, Inner Thigh Lifts,* and *Outer Thigh Lifts* for ten lifts per movement per leg. Repeat for the other side.

7. Come to standing and feel five breaths in *Awkward Chair Pose.*

8. Follow with five breaths in *Pulsing Squats* with *PFCR*.

9. Come to the floor into *Cow Face Pose* with a side bend. Feel eight breaths per side.

10. Come into *Cobbler's Pose* for eight breaths.

11. Bring your legs long into *Staff Pose* and slowly fold forward using a strap for *Seated Forward Fold* for five breaths.

12. Come into *Seated Wide-Legged Forward Fold Pose* for five breaths.
13. Lie back and feel five breaths in *Bridge Pose*. Repeat once or twice more.
14. Come into *Legs Up the Wall Pose* for five minutes.
15. End your practice with five minutes of *Rest and Relaxation Pose*.

Embodied Vocal Exploration: Sanskrit Chanting

Whenever you have little time for a *Movement-Based Practice*, a short chanting and meditation session can do wonders to restore your energy.

Below are some *mantras* and chants I share with my students for centering and meditation. They all create opportunities to free the voice, feel vocal vibration resonating in the skull, and center you for meditation. You can find recordings of these chants on my website www.melissahurt.com/chants.

OM

You can find *OM* spelled two ways: *OM* and *AUM*. The second spelling reveals more of the phonetic experience of the sound. *OM* represents the sound of Divinity. Every time we chant *OM*, it's as if we are connecting to God by not only saying his name but also sounding the vibration of which He is the pure essence.

There are four parts to *OM*—three are sounded, and the last is silent. Begin *OM* by first inhaling; you inspire yourself for connection. Next, open your mouth to the #5 vowel lip opening, the most comfortable lip opening you can make without unhinging your jaw. You will vocalize AH. This sound starts in the back of your mouth, and you may feel it resonates in your solar plexus. As you move the lips toward the #1 lip opening (the U in *AUM*), the vocal vibrations will resonate from the back of the mouth along the ridge of the hard palate until you arrive at the smallest circle you can comfortably make with your lips—the #1. You may feel the sound resonate in the throat.

Next, close the lips to a comfortable M and feel the vibrations on the lips waft up into the sinus cavity, the third eye in between the eyebrows, and then perhaps the crown of the head. Last, finish the vocalization at the base of your exhalation, enjoy the silence, and feel the residual vibrations.

The vibrations that linger, the fourth part of the *OM*, are just as important as the three sounded parts—A, U, M. Feel the four parts of this chant again as often as you like. The more you chant *OM*, the greater you can connect with your full, open, rich voice as it vibrates in your body. This act is both grounding and uplifting at once.

Some prefer to chant *OM* with a #21 vowel—OH—and an M. This is fine, too. If you feel a true circular lip opening on the #21 vowel with a yawn-like sensation in the back of the mouth, you will be able to feel the vocal vibrations of the vowel resonate at the center of the cathedral of the hard palate and through the crown of the head. This also creates a focal point for meditation and opens the crown for your connection to Divinity.

Chant *OM* several times in a row. Notice how your baby lights up when you chant it. I have *never* seen a baby *not* find stillness for several moments when I chant *OM* with the postnatal yoga class. It is truly magical. *OM* is a powerful chant and meditative tool. It allows you to connect with yourself, your baby, and the Divine within and all around.

Lokah Samastah Sukino Bhavantu

Don't be intimidated by Sanskrit, the ancient language of yoga. It is a language with rich musicality that feels wonderful to speak. The tactile nature of Sanskrit vibrates at different points along the length of the hard palate and lips, centering the meditator into a relaxing, yet uplifting, chanting session. A popular chant is **Lokah Samastah Sukino Bhavantu**, meaning "May all beings be happy and free, and may all thoughts, words, and actions of my own life contribute in some way to that happiness and to that freedom for all."[29]

The ways to pronounce and feel the sounds of this chant are as follows:

Lokah—the first vowel is a #21 and the second vowel is a #5. The H at the end of the word is a small aspiration. The word feels like "LOH-KAH-ha."

Samastah—all three vowels are #5 vowels. The H at the end of the word is a small aspiration (as in "ha"). The word feels like "SAH-MAH-STAH-ha."

Sukino—the first vowel is a #1, the second vowel is a Y buzz, and the last vowel is a #21. The Y buzz in Sukino is a short Y buzz, as in the second syllable of "simply." The word feels like "Soo-KEE-NOH."

Bhavantu—the first vowel is a #5, the second vowel is a #5, and the last vowel is a #1. The H after the B is a small aspiration (breath) into the #5 vowel in the first syllable. The word feels like "B(h)AH—VAH—Too."

The consonants in this chant feel as they would in English. You can enjoy the humming vibrations in the N in *Bhavantu* to a moment of tactile grounding. Be sure to keep the aspirations of the H small as they appear.

Now string it all together:
LOH-KAH-ha SAH-MAH-STAH-ha Soo-KEE-NOH B(h)AH—VAH—Too

Lokah Samastah Sukino Bhavantu
You can chant this *mantra* as many times as you like to feel peaceful and grounded. The more you connect with the sounds and meaning of the chant, the more you will positively affect your surroundings with the message of the chant: *sending peace, freedom, and happiness to the world, starting with those immediately around you.*

Om shanti, shanti, shanti

Shanti means "peace" so when we chant "*Om, shanti, shanti, shanti,*" we are connecting to the Divine within and around us and sending peace for ourselves and the world. "*Om, shanti, shanti, shanti*" popularly ends a chant to finalize our intentions for the vibrations that wafted through the crowns of our heads into the heavens.

I personally love this chant because it opens my mouth fully and takes me back to a grounded Y buzz at the end of each "*shanti.*" In "*shanti,*" the first syllable is a #5 vowel, and the second syllable is a Y buzz. When we chant the phrase, we go up in pitch on the final Y buzz, then back down a half pitch. We typically close the chanting with a resounding *OM.*

You can feel the fullness of the chant by exploring these directions:

Inhale
On *exhale,* chant:
OM, ShAHn-TEE, ShAHn-TEE, ShAHn-TEE
Inhale
OM

Feel this *OM* for as long as your exhalation and let the vibrations in silence carry into the ether. Many yogis popularly put this chant at the end of **Lokah Samastah Sukino Bhavantu.**

You can feel them together in this way:
Inhale
Exhale on:
OM Lokah Samastah Sukino Bhavantu
Inhale
Lokah Samastah Sukino Bhavantu
Inhale
Lokah Samastah Sukino Bhavantu

Inhale
OM Shanti, Shanti, Shanti
Inhale
Exhale on:
OM
Silent meditation.
(It's okay to take mini-inhalations between the words if you need to.)

Atha yoganushasanam

At times, yogis like to chant lines from the *Yoga Sutras*, the ancient text recorded by Patañjali that describes the many observances and codes of yoga that bring one to full absorption with the Divine within and beyond. There are 196 sutras, or rules, and any of them can be used for chanting meditation if you know how to read and feel the Sanskrit language.

The first *yoga sutra* is accessible and a popular choice. When not listed with the traditional Sanskrit diacritical markings, it reads "*Atha yoganushasanam*" and translates to "Now, the teaching of yoga."[30] Some scholars prefer to read into this and pronounce it as if were declaring the present moment: "NOW, the teaching of yoga begins. It all starts NOW. Be present and pay attention!" Instead, it simply states that the lesson of yoga is beginning like how a stylized letter symbolized the start of a book section hundreds of years ago. That said, it *is* nice to acknowledge that something is beginning. The interesting part is in what follows—the path, the unfolding, and the evolution of self.

We feel "*atha yoganushasanam*" as follows:
Atha—The first syllable is a #5 and the second begins with a T consonant, a tiny aspiration on
the H and a #5 vowel. It feels like "AH-T(h)AH."
Yoga—The first syllable is a #21 vowel, and the second syllable is a #5 vowel. It feels like "YOH-GAH."

Nusha—The first syllable is a #1 vowel, and the second syllable begins with an SH consonant (as if quieting your baby) and a #5 vowel. It feels like "Nooo-ShAH."

Sanam—Both syllables are a #5 vowel. It feels like "SAH-NAHM." You can enjoy the hum of the M at the end of "sanam."

Put it together slowly with mindfulness of the rhythm of it all:

Inhale

AH-T(h)AH YOH-GAH Nooo-ShAH SAH-NAHM

Then again, stringing it together a bit more:

Inhale

AH-T(h)AH YOH-GAH Nooo-ShAH SAH-NAHM

Then put it all together:

Inhale

AH-T(h)AH YOH-GAHNooo-ShAHSAH-NAHM

AthaYoga nusha sanam

Atha Yoganushasanam

Spend time with these chants and discover which one is your favorite.

Meditation: Chant Chakra Scan

Chant your favorite chant from the *Embodied Voice Exploration* above continuously for two to four minutes. Then go through the *Chakra Scan* meditation while feeling the vocal vibration as a part of your energetic scan and grounding.

Optional: Read about *surrender* in **Part Four** and journal what you discover about this practice. I encourage you to continue your exploration of this principle as you move through the program.

Summary

Congratulations, you did it! By now, you are stronger and steadier in your joints. You have explored a range of *Breath-Based Practices* to discover myriad ways to find calm focus and clarity of body, mind, and spirit. You have found and developed your embodied voice. You are connected with the tactile feeling of the inside of your mouth, the feeling of your breath, and how it becomes your vocal life. The voice expresses your truths, your fears, your wishes, and your needs to connect. When you speak with a resonant, vibrating, and warm voice, you embrace the richness of your vocal life as you authentically recognize your emotional and spiritual self. You can incorporate *Embodied Voice Practices* in your daily life whenever you speak to another, read a book to your baby, or sing in the shower or the car. The more you enjoy the feeling of your voice, the more energy you will receive from your body, mind, breath, and spirit at once.

I encourage you to hold loving-kindness toward your intention in your *Movement-Based Practices* to fully engage with your whole self as you work to achieve balanced and vital wellness in your life. As with any yoga practice, the more you create kindness and love for yourself on the mat, the more you will continue to do so off the mat. And the more you take care of yourself in this manner, the better you can take care of others. The better they respond to the positivity you bring to them, the better you will feel. It all synergizes and grows from there. I suggest adding a *mantra* or chant to your daily *Meditation Practice* at least twice a week to deepen your connection with yourself and the Divine.

You can circle back to **Phase One** and repeat the program again and again. When you do, you will continue to get stronger, more flexible, and more balanced and stable. You will discover qualities of your voice again and again as you develop enriching vocal dynamics for a vibrant vocal life. As your child gets older and your life moves through different seasons, your *Meditation Practice* will be a touchstone to your Divine self. You are centered. You have found your inner space that is your source of peace and your Divine light. It is there for you whenever you need it.

If you have started the program in your first year postpartum, but have yet to reach your child's first birthday, I advise repeating

Part Two once more until you reach this milestone. This is to ensure you are healing diastasis recti and stabilizing your hips and core safely in preparation for **Phase Seven** in **Part Three**. If you are starting this program with a child that is older than one-year-old, please start at the beginning of **Part Two** so you can use the range of practices as an entryway to self-study. You will build strength, flexibility, and balance through these gentle yet effective practices that can better prepare you for the next phase of the program.

~ 4 ~

PART THREE: RESTORATION
BEYOND THE FIRST YEAR

Many mothers feel like their child's first birthday is a significant triumph for both baby *and* mama. You've made it past the exhaustion of the fourth trimester, worked through sleep regressions, worked through the baby cutting teeth, trialed foods to determine which your baby can digest well, baby-proofed the house once your scooter becomes a crawler, and perhaps done *more* baby-proofing once that baby discovers walking can turn into running! It's a time filled with joy, fatigue, curiosity, and wonder.

You have completed the six-phase program and feel more integrated with body, mind, voice, and spirit. Hopefully, you have repeated the program at least once to build stability, spiritual clarity, and vocal warmth and power. You are stepping into a strong sense of self that is free and dynamic at once. It's a beautiful process!

Hopefully, by the time you start your second year postpartum (once your baby turns one year old), you will sleep more, eat better, and maintain relationships with other mothers. You are certainly moving more to keep up with your child! You are now in **Phase Seven**, which has three more weeks of *Breath-Based Practices*, stronger *Movement-Based Practices*, more advanced *Embodied Voice Practices*, and *Meditations*. Consider it *The Postpartum Path of Yoga version 2.0*.

I include lunges and kneeling planks at this part of the program to explore regaining dynamic flexibility and strength in the muscles surrounding the pelvis. If you spent time stabilizing the pelvis through the six phases thus far and have explored them over the first year postpartum, you will be ready to hold lunges, standing lunges safely, and Warrior poses. The yoga *asana* practice gets stronger at this phase so you can begin to recapture more of the vitality you may have felt pre-pregnancy. In addition, I include kneeling planks that evolve into full planks once the front of the core feels strong and stable to support the lower back. Lastly, I include some poses, such as *Boat Pose* and poses from mat Pilates abdominal series, that specifically target strengthening the abdominal muscles. Only perform these poses when you have determined you have corrected diastasis recti.

You will continue pelvic floor contraction and release exercises daily—let these be a component of self-care that is as normal and regular as brushing your teeth. As your body changes over time, you will be thankful you kept these up. Trust me, your sixty-year-old self thanks you! Continue growing your community. Share these practices with others. Laugh often. Enjoy your child and let them see you doing these practices. The sooner you model self-care, the more they will learn that they are capable of self-regulation and self-care. Besides, you show them that Mama is important and needs to nurture herself to take care of the family. Lastly, let your meditation practice be a compass for your spiritual life. A daily practice of even five minutes daily will keep you connected to your spiritual alignment and inner voice. This becomes important not just for spiritual growth over a lifetime, but for recognizing how your values resonate with you when you need to make choices for yourself and your family. Trust yourself, but first, you need to get to know yourself.

We frame the work in **Phase Seven** with excerpts from the *Bhagavad Gita*, the classic spiritual tale of Lord Krishna teaching Arjuna, the prized warrior, how to find and step into his *dharma* through the act of yoga. Arjuna struggles with his core sense of self as he faces battle, and Krishna educates him on his duty to serve and live his life as an act of service to Him, the Supreme Lord. He teaches meditation is the best way to do this while finding your true self. The more you learn the ways of yoga, the more you become balanced in your mind and aligned with God within. Additionally, He teaches the importance of service with complete non-attachment to results. Instead, find God in the act itself. The *Bhagavad Gita* is a book to read yearly as a self-inquiry guideline. I include three small excerpts from the text as a frame for the next three weeks and encourage you to find a copy of this sacred text and use it to discover yourself on a deeper level.

A note about religion: you are not defying your faith or commitment to your religion if you learn from the *Bhagavad Gita*. Many faiths share the same principles, and I think you will find many commonalities between these teachings and what you hold true in your heart about God, personal integrity, and finding your calling. Moreover, if you do not connect with the name "God," please replace it with whatever energy greater than yourself that lifts you to a better place, be it the Universe, the Holy Spirit, or Magic. It is all the same force, just assigned a different name.

We are all Arjuna as he finds himself at the story's beginning: agitated, confused and not wanting to hurt others through our actions. If you dedicate yourself to yoga and meditation, you arrive at your true self, find the Work that is meant for you, and choose practices that nourish yourself in body, mind, and spirit.

Phase Seven, Week One

Better is [one's] own-law imperfectly [carried out] than another's law well-performed. Performing the action necessitated by [one's] own-being, [the yogin] does not accumulate guilt.

Bhagavad Gita 18.47

The "law" Krishna speaks of is your calling. Find the action, the thing, the Work, you are meant to do, and do it the best you know how. What is that, and how do you find it? It's the work you do when time disappears, you feel completely aligned in body, mind, and spirit, and you feel light doing it. This is your groove. It is your dharmic law to perform this the most honest way you know how. Doing work that meets an assumed standard but feel strained or difficult spiritually is not in your best interest, even if you do it amazingly well. Instead, be true to yourself and don't strive to act in ways true to others. If you copy others, you are not being authentic and take on implicit guilt for not being your best self. Meditate on this. Get still and quiet and ask, "When am I feeling most like myself? When am I most free? What am I doing in these moments?" and notice what comes.

Breath-Based Practice: Reclined Skull-Shining Breath, *Kapalabhati*

This breathing practice is known as the "breath of fire." It detoxifies the body and tones the internal organs at the abdomen due to its pump-like action. Some feel the oxygenation of the practice clarifies their energy all over. *Caution: Do not perform this breath if you are pregnant, menstruating, have heart complications, or have high blood pressure. You will want to wait two hours after eating to perform this breathing practice.*

Begin by lying in a semi-supine position with the spine long and relaxed. Feel your lower belly drawing inwards as you exhale and let the inhalation happen naturally. Stay here for as long as you like to feel the action of the lower belly. Next, increase the momentum of the exhalations such that the lower belly pushes air out very quickly. Mini-inhalations will happen naturally. You will feel a purposeful and robust inward pump of the low belly with air moving out of the nostrils. Your belly will not completely release on the inhalations. Explore the exhalation pumping for one minute, then return to natural breathing for a couple of minutes. Repeat two or three more times. End with relaxed natural breathing and notice the energy this practice has given you.

Movement-Based Practice: Find Your Feet Supporting You
This week, we will modify the sequence from **Phase Six, Week Three**. Remain aware of the synchronization of the breath and the deep core muscles.

1. Begin in *Table Pose* and flow from *Cow Pose* to *Cat Pose* on the rhythm of your breath while also engaging PFCR. Feel ten of these flows as you inhale in *Cow Pose* (relax the pelvic floor) and exhale in *Cat Pose* (contract the pelvic floor).
2. Move into *Bird Dog Pose* and add *spinal flexion* on the exhalation.
3. Come onto your belly for the flow in starting and ending with *Locust Pose*. Complete four repetitions.
4. Come into *Kneeling Plank Pose:*

Kneeling Plank

- Come to *Table Pose* with your hands directly under your shoulders.
- Engage your abdominal muscles towards your spine, but do not suck the belly in. You want to breathe naturally.

- Walk the knees back to where you can feel your spine as a long line of energy.
- Tilt the pelvis such that you feel the pubic bone moving towards your nose and tailbone pointing more towards the hollows of your knees. You will feel the front of the trunk engage.
- Keep your gaze between your hands so the crown of your head is in line with the rest of the spine. You will feel length throughout the spine while honoring the natural curves inward of the neck and lower back. Breathe here for five breaths.

5. Come into *Extended Child's Pose* for five breaths.

6. Come onto your left side for *Modified Side Plank* for eight breaths.

7. Come to standing and feel five breaths in *Awkward Chair Pose*.

8. Come into *Tall Crescent Lunge Pose:*

Tall Crescent Lunge Pose

- Begin in *Mountain Pose.*
- Step your left foot back and step onto the ball of the foot keeping the heel up.
- Bend the right knee as much as you are able while also engaging your energy through the left leg and into the ball of the foot. This will stabilize you.
- Raise up the arms long and engage your energy through your fingers. *Caution: If you have high blood pressure, you will want to skip this part and keep your hands on your hips.*
- Stay here for five breaths. Return to *Mountain Pose* and repeat with the right foot back.

9. Bring your legs long into *Staff Pose* and slowly fold forward using a strap for *Seated Forward Fold* for five breaths.

10. Come to the floor into *Cow Face Pose* with a side bend. Feel eight breaths per side.

11. Come into *Cobbler's Pose* for eight breaths.

12. Lie back and feel five breaths in *Bridge Pose*. Repeat once or twice more.

13. Explore *Pelvic Floor Contraction and Relaxation* (PFCR) exercises while sitting upright and finding an *optimal postural alignment* of pelvis, ribs, and head.

14. Come into *Legs Up the Wall Pose* for five minutes.

15. End your practice with five minutes of *Rest and Relaxation Pose*.

Embodied Voice Exploration: The + Y Buzz

The + Y Buzz expands your awareness of your vocal power and strength without feeling any pain or strain in your voice. You will develop more vocal warmth and resonance with this practice.

- Begin by feeling a comfortable Y Buzz in the lower third of your speaking range.

A few reminders:

- Sustain the reverse megaphone forward facial orientation and breathe comfortably.
- Feel the Y consonant with a true long E vowel
- Smile in your eyes (remember, we want engaged behavior)
- Feel a sense of floating through the crown of your head
- Massage the Y buzz with a gentle pulse: "Yeee—yeee-yeee-yeee-yeee."
  Keep breathing naturally; there's no need to push your breath through any of this work.
- Now sustain the space in your mouth and change the long E vowel to a long A vowel—"yeeee" becomes "yay." Do not move your jaw to feel this—keep the shape of the reverse megaphone intact.

- Pulse the + Y Buzz—"yay" "yay" "yay." You will feel a larger ping of vocal resonance that meets the upper gum ridge and the space of the hard palate just ahead of it as your awareness moves along the roof of the mouth.
- Explore the words: **baby, lazy, made, shade, late, escapade, today.** You will feel the ping of the + Y Buzz on the long A vowels in these words and the ping of the Y Buzz on the long E vowels (where appropriate).

Meditation: The Space In-Between Breaths

A teaching I share with all my students is finding the stillness at the center of your being. You can notice it if you tend to the pauses at the seat of every inhalation and every exhalation. We tend to focus more on the intake of breath and sharing the exhalation with the surrounding air. More interesting, though, is the natural pauses that happen after these events. It's like your body is telling you, "Wait. Stop. Notice. See what I just gave you? No, not the breath...the window to see yourself. Right. Now."

This meditation broadens your awareness to your access within. Take time to be curious about yourself and your process. Find patience. This will slow your breathing rhythm to its natural, optimal flow. Once you feel stillness, explore staying with it while still breathing.

To begin, sit comfortably and focus on the movement of your breath. You can revisit "pleasure smelling" from **Phase One, Week One** to recall a natural way to receive an optimal breath. There is a natural pause at the seat of your inhalation. Notice your suspension in this space while also feeling grounded in your seat. Exhale slowly. Notice the feeling of buoyancy once you arrive at the pause at the end of exhalation. Keep breathing and focus with loving kindness on the spaces between inhalation and exhalation. Your true self lies within these moments.

Phase Seven, Week Two

He [whose] self is yoked through Yoga [and who] everywhere beholds the same [vision of sameness amongst all beings] sees the Self abiding in all beings and all beings in the Self. He who sees Me everywhere and sees all in Me, to him I am not lost, nor is he lost to Me. He who is established in oneness [and] worships Me abiding in all beings, howsoever indeed he exists—that yogin dwells in Me.
Bhagavad Gita 6.29-6.31

The eight-limbed practice of yoga, including breathing practices, mindful movements (*asana*), and meditation, brings the practitioner to experience God within. You have felt this by this stage of your path! Krishna teaches that when we feel God inside of ourselves, we recognize He is everywhere. There is something very grounding and calming in this. God is with you always, and you can feel His presence with every breath, movement, and look inward. We treat our neighbors, the citizens of the world, and the environment with more kindness and are more receptive to them when we feel in our hearts that they are no different from us on a heart-mind level. We are of universal consciousness, and we all seek peace. Keeping on the yogic pathway tills the soil of the spirit so we can receive our gifts and share them with others. If everyone lived life this way, how beautiful would the world be!

Breath-Based Practice: Seated Skull-Shining Breath

Last week we explored *Skull-Shining Breath* in a reclined position. This week we will be upright in a chair or seated on a folded blanket or cushion. In this orientation, you will feel a boost in the energy radiating up through the crown of the head.

Find a tall spine as you sit. You can bow your head a bit to engage a yogic chin lock, which will help to focus your energy inward.

Place your hands on your lower belly and explore the pumping exhalation from last week. Take time to feel the inward and upward draw of the lower belly. Relax for thirty seconds. Once you have determined you have this action, perform the quick *Skull-Shining Breath* for one minute. Relax for two minutes. Repeat two to three times with two minutes of relaxation after each round. Notice the lift in your energy!

Movement-Based Practice: Grounded Strength, Light Heart
We will revisit lengthening the side body to open our awareness of spaciousness through the trunk as we move into strong standing poses.

1. Begin in *Extended Child's Pose*. Lengthen your spine with each breath. Stay here for five to eight breaths.
2. Come into *Table Pose* and flow in *Bird Dog Pose*. Explore five repetitions from balancing with alternating the right arm/ left leg and left arm/right leg. Keep your abdominal muscles engaged towards the spine to protect the lower back.
3. Come into *Modified Side Plank*. Focus on the length of the sides of the body as you breathe for eight breaths per side.
4. Come into *Kneeling Plank* or explore *Full Plank*. To come into *Full Plank*, begin in *Kneeling Plank* and extend one leg out at a time while coming onto the balls of the feet. If you feel your hips dropping towards the floor or a pull in your mid-to-low back, come back to *Kneeling Plank*. Breathe here for eight breaths.
5. Come into Table Pose and bring your right foot forward for *Runner's Lunge:*

Runner's Lunge

• Ground your energy through your right foot while extending your left leg back. Come onto the ball of the left foot.

- Keep your breastbone lengthening towards the space ahead so you do not collapse at the chest. We want to feel length of the sides of the body. Place your hands on tall yoga blocks to assist with this action.
- Breathe here for five breaths while focusing on extending energy through the left leg while also lengthening the breastbone forwards and up.
- Come back to *Table Pose* and change sides for five breaths.

6. Come into *Mountain Pose*. Explore five *Half Sun Salutations*.

7. Return to *Mountain Pose* and explore *Warrior 1:*

Warrior 1, Virabhadrasana I

- Step the left foot back and pivot on the ball of the foot so the whole foot can engage into the ground. Do not worry if your hips face a little more to the left.
- Bend your right knee while also engaging your awareness through the left foot. Be aware if you are collapsing the inner arch. If so, engage more in the mound beneath the big toe, the mound beneath the pinky toe, and the center of the heel.
- Lift your arms up and extend energy through your fingers. Your palms will face each other. You can bring your hands together if you do not have any neck or shoulder tension. You will feel a slight back bend at the upper-to-mid back. *Caution: if you have high blood pressure, you will keep your hands on your hips.* Breathe here for five breaths.
- Bring the arms down and step the left foot forward. Repeat with the right foot back for five breaths.

8. Come to *Staff Pose* for five breaths. Explore *Twisted Staff Pose* for five breaths on each side.

9. Explore *Modified Boat Pose:*

Modified Boat Pose, *Navasana*

- Sit on your sitting bones with your legs bent and balls of feet on the ground. Hold behind the thighs.
- Lengthen through the crown of the head, focusing on lengthening the breastbone up to keep the chest from collapsing.
- Bring your feet up, keeping your shins parallel to the ceiling.
- Lean back a bit to engage the core while breathing optimally. If you feel strong here, you can release the backs of the thighs and extend the arms around your shins.
- Breathe here for five to eight complete breaths. Bring your feet down and hug your knees to release.

10. Come to *Bridge Pose* for eight breaths. Repeat once or twice more with a nice rest in
between.

11. Explore pelvic tilts with *PFCR* for ten to fifteen breath cycles.

12. Relax in *Rest and Relaxation Pose* for five to ten minutes.

Embodied Voice Exploration: The Call

This vocal exploration continues your connection with your personal power through your voice. Remember to ease into your voice and do not push or force. The Call develops your vocal range and is the bridge to embodied, connected singing!

- Begin by feeling a Y Buzz.
- Let the Y Buzz evolve into the + Y Buzz, remembering to sustain the reverse megaphone.
- Create an intention O shape of the lips and change the long A vowel to a long O vowel as you say "h'llO!" or "Yo!." Stay on the same pitch you had for the + Y Buzz and focus on the expansion of your vocal energy on the roof of your mouth.

- Feeling the "O" vowel, explore the roundness of the lips forward, the forward movement of the check muscles and the openness at the back of the throat to create a more extravagant reverse megaphone. Begin to go up one pitch saying/chanting either "h'llO!" or "Yo!" with your upwards movement on the long O vowel.
- Explore moving up in pitch no more than three pitches until you move into the mid-Call range. You will feel you need to enlarge the circular lip opening to track the resonance of the Call on the hard palate. If you do not, you will not feel the vibration on the hard palate. Awareness of this vibration is key, so you do not resort to shouting.
- Return to a gentle Y Buzz and then hum on an M. Breathe easily and enjoy the effects of these powerful vocal vibrations.

Meditation: Observe Your Thoughts Passing By

People popularly think meditation is about emptying your mind and becoming an empty vessel for the divine spirit. This is not true! It is impossible to empty the mind because we are always sensing, emoting, and thinking. Our brains are active, which is good. If they were not active, then we would be dead!

Working to empty the mind of thoughts will only bring on tension due to the impossibility of the task. You can, though, become an observer of your thoughts. You can regard as Sally Kempton, a respected meditation teacher, does as if they are clouds in the sky. Often when I meditate and a stream of thoughts about my to-do list enters, I watch the thoughts scroll by like ticker tape on the TV news. I then say, "That's fine, but I can tend to you later," and I instantly return to my breath awareness.

Try this: find a comfortable seat and close your eyes. Become aware of your breathing: how the body expands and contrasts upon its entry and departure, how its temperature feels in your nose coming and going, and its rate of inhalation and exhalation. Notice any thoughts that enter and observe them passing by like clouds in the sky.[31] You do not get lost in them. You watch them come and go while you keep your awareness on your breath.

Phase Seven, Week Three

Hear again My supreme word, most secret of all. You are thus surely beloved of Me. Therefore, I will tell you [wherein lies your] welfare. Be Me-minded, devoted to Me, sacrifice to Me, make reverence to Me—thus you will come to Me. I promise you truly, [for] you are dear to Me.
Bhagavad Gita 18.64-18.65

These verses loop back to my initial message to you via *Yoga Sutra* 1.20: the pathway to restoring yourself begins with faith in something bigger than yourself. If we incorporate the *Bhagavad Gita*, we can call that God. This verse tells us that God is with us because He loves us. Part of our work is to hold this in your heart, take care of yourself, and serve Him in how you treat others. I promise you that when you open your heart to this idea and share your gifts with others, abundance will manifest for you. It may not be monetary wealth, but you will find abundant energy, vitality, love, kindness, patience, creativity, and community support and respect. I'd take any or all of those over a larger bank account any day! Find comfort in how cherished and valuable you are. Taking care of yourself means you honor the body, mind, and voice God gave you so you can grow in spirit and share your *dharma* with the world. You got this.

Breath-Based Practice: The Cooling Breaths, *Sitali Pranayama*
These breathing practices cool the body and mind, moisturize the body, and reduce fatigue. They are lovely to do whenever you feel stressed, agitated, or hot (especially on summer days!). There are two options for the *Cooling Breath*: curling the side of the tongue

up to create a straw-like shape or keeping the upper and lower teeth together for those who cannot curl the tongue. For those curling the tongue, protrude the tongue out of the mouth about three-quarters of an inch. Both ways have a cooling effect.

Begin by either curling the tongue or keeping the teeth together, lips apart. Inhale through this space. Bring the lips together (and retract the tongue in) and exhale through the nose. Close your eyes as you explore this breathing practice to keep your awareness inwards. Repeat your inhalations with the lips apart and either protruding your curled tongue or inhaling through the teeth. Exhale with lips together. Repeat this practice for two to three minutes. Return to natural breathing and notice its effect.

Movement-Based Practice: Inner and Outer Strength Radiating Outward

This practice will integrate many of the stronger poses from the program while cooling down nicely into a beautiful rest in which you can feel your inner power shining through.

1. Begin with five *Half Sun Salutations*, including *Extended Puppy Dog Pose*. If you feel strong in your abdomen and back, straighten the legs for a full expression of *Downward Facing Dog Pose*. Enjoy five breaths in each *Extended Puppy Dog* or *Downward Facing Dog Pose*.
2. Come into *Kneeling Plank Pose* or *Full Plank Pose* for five breaths. Rest in *Extended Child's Pose* for a few moments, then repeat.
3. Come into *Mountain Pose,* then into *Awkward Chair Pose* for five breaths. Repeat twice.
4. Step the left leg back for either Tall Crescent Lunge Pose or Warrior 1 Pose. Focus on the strength you feel in your legs, the length in your trunk, and the openness across the chest. Enjoy each pose for five breaths. Return to Mountain Pose then change sides for five breaths.

5. Step your feet wide into *Goddess Pose*. Add a dynamic flow by *inhaling* as you draw the arms up with your legs straight. *Exhale*, and draw the arms into a goalpost shape while bending the knees. Engage the bottom tips of the shoulder blades together. Repeat this flow on your natural breath rhythm four more times.

6. Come into *Standing Forward Fold Pose* for three to five breaths.

7. Come into *Extended Puppy Dog Pose* or *Downward Facing Dog Pose* for five breaths.

8. Bring the right foot forward for *Runner's Lunge Pose*. Breathe here for five breaths. Return to *Extended Puppy Dog Pose* or *Downward Facing Dog Pose* and bring the left foot forward for *Runner's Lunge Pose*. Breathe here for five breaths. Return to *Extended Puppy Dog Pose* or *Downward Facing Dog Pose*.

9. Come into *Staff Pose* and slowly fold forward using a strap for *Seated Forward Fold* for five breaths.

10. Come into *Cow Face Pose* with a side bend. Feel eight breaths per side.

11. Come into *Modified Boat Pose* for five to eight breaths. Rest for a moment, then repeat.

12. Come into *Cobbler's Pose* for eight breaths.

13. Lie back and feel five breaths in *Bridge Pose*. Repeat once or twice more.

14. Explore *Pelvic Floor Contraction and Relaxation* (PFCR) exercises while sitting upright and finding an *optimal postural alignment* of the pelvis, ribs, and head.

15. End your practice with five minutes of *Rest and Relaxation Pose*.

Embodied Voice Exploration: Track the Call to Harness Your Power

Now that you have felt your low Call, you can develop its power and range by tracking it up three pitches into your mid-Call range. This practice further develops your vocal power without any pain and brings you into a state of trusting your bodymind's capacity to create the shape and space with your mouth that your voice needs to come forth. Similarly, discover how you can create the space you need to thrive. Sometimes we get in our way by trying to do too much. Instead, can you provide the essentials and let the process take over?

- Begin by humming on a Y Buzz (yeee...yeee...yeee)
- Bring the Y Buzz into the + Y Buzz (yay...yay...yay...). You will have the same size reverse megaphone for each.
- Now feel a low Call on "YO!" or "H'llO!" by creating a circular lip opening and feeling more yawn in the back of the throat. The vocal resonance will take up more surface area on the hard palate.
- Once you feel a low Call, you will open your awareness to how you sustain the vibration on your hard palate while bringing the pitch up one note. You will feel a "YOOOOOO!" and go up one note on the long O vowel. Notice if you need to make subtle shifts to the reverse megaphone to keep the vibration on the roof of the mouth. Keep it on this pitch.
- Next, begin the Call on this slightly higher pitch and go up one more pitch on the long O vowel as you did in the last step. Again, you are at the service of the Call. Let your bodymind show you how to subtly negotiate the yawn space in the back of the throat to accommodate the higher pitch. Keep it on this pitch.
- Lastly, Call again on this pitch and you will take it up one more pitch, so long as you feel as if you are comfortable and not pushing or straining *at all*. You may have a larger circular lip opening by this point—this is fine. Explore what your reverse megaphone shape needs to become to hone vibration on the roof of the mouth.

- To end the exploration, return to a + Y Buzz and then to a comfortable Y Buzz. Your voice should feel rich, warm, and vibrant with zero strain in the throat.

Meditation: Loving Kindness for All (Yourself, Loved Ones, Strangers, Difficult People, All Beings)

It seems obvious to express loving kindness to those we love. Whether we explicitly share our love and gratitude with our families, we certainly find ways to express our feelings through hugs, kind notes, or quick phone calls. Sometimes, we need help discovering what true loving kindness is and how we are meant to share it with everyone. You might think, "What about the people who aggravate me? What about total strangers?" Yes, I say, all people deserve love.

Once you open yourself to a non-discriminatory level of loving-kindness, you find you have much more to give energetically and are more receptive to others' love and gratitude towards yourself.

To begin: find a comfortable seat and become aware of your breath.

- Cultivate loving kindness for yourself with the *mantras*:
  - May I be filled with loving-kindness.
  - May I be safe from inner and outer dangers.
  - May I be well in body and mind.
  - May I be at ease and happy.[32]
- Open your heart to fully receive these messages. Breathe them in. Honor them in yourself. Take your time with this.
- Next, send these messages to the following people (changing the "I" to "you"), taking time with each:
  - A beloved person in your life
  - A person who is difficult in your life.
  - Someone you pass in your daily life, but do not engage with.

- Next, broaden your awareness to your neighborhood and send the message to your neighbors. Then broaden it to your town. Next, your state. Next, your country. Next, the entire world. Hold the world in your awareness and send the message to all citizens in the world. If you want to go further, express loving kindness to all animals and to the environment.
- Sit, breathe, hold these spaces and people in your heart. Imagine they all send the messages of loving kindness back to you. Breathe here feeling the love for as long as you like.

Summary

You have now explored stronger practices to dive more deeply into your personal power physically, vocally, and spiritually. Continue to explore these practices alone or in conjunction with those in Phases One through Six. You may feel more tired some days and will want to keep your daily practice to breath-based awareness, meditation, and foundational movements from **Phase One**. On other days you can spend the bulk of your time exploring a range of embodied voice practices. On days in which you feel more vigor, you want to create a personal practice out of **Phase One** through **Phase Six** and spend more time on three of the standing lunges in **Phase Seven**. As you can see from my examples, you have the freedom to craft what best serves you. *The Postpartum Path of Yoga* has taught you many skills to learn about yourself. You continually discover what practices create strength, relaxation, and inner peace as you grow as a woman and mother. Return to them often and enjoy the magic of cultivating self-care rituals that best serve you. Share your ideas with the friends you have found through the community prompts. Create a meet-up in which you practice together and support one another. The possibilities for your growth and evolution are endless.

~ 5 ~

PART FOUR: CONNECTING WITH OTHERS, LOVING YOURSELF

According to the *Yoga Sutras*, we have an eight-limbed path to the practice and life of yoga. The first limb is the *yamas*, and the second is the niyamas, the yoga practitioner's guidelines for interactions with others (the *yamas*) and personal behavior (the *niyamas*).[33] Think of the *yamas* as the ethical practices for being in this world and the *niyamas* as the best codes for self-care for discovering and preserving your best self. This section includes a teaching on each guideline and questions for reflection. I have included the name of each observance in Sanskrit in parenthesis after its introduction for you to refer to in case you want further research on these observances.

Think of the *yamas* as the ethical practices for being in this world and the *niyamas* as the best codes for self-care for discovering and preserving your best self.

The Yamas: Connecting with Others

These ethical codes teach how to relate to other people. You would apply these principles as questions to how you inhabit the earth and engage with others. You can also dig deeper and ask how you relate to yourself.

The *yamas* make up the first limb of the eight-limbed path of yoga because we can determine how effective our practice is based on how we treat others. You may have felt this in your personal life. When you are quick to snap at your child over a small matter, don't you notice how you usually are not feeling well in body, mind, and spirit? Are you quick to judge? Do you grow angry easily? Do you speak to others dishonestly, even tell little "white lies"? As Nicholai Bachman teaches, "The way we treat other living creatures is a testament to our inner state. Clarity in our heart-mind manifests as kindness, compassion, selflessness, keen judgment, etc. Cloudiness reveals itself as malice, selfishness, poor judgment, etc."[34]

I encourage you to dig deeply into the *yamas* and be honest with what you find. Keep a journal to record your reflections, questions, and musings. Respect yourself with kindness and without judgment. The real work of yoga begins here.

NON-HARMING

Non-harming (*ahimsā*) is the first of the *yamas* that starts you on your path. *Non-harming* includes restraining violence in thought, words, and actions against people, animals, and the environment. It's not difficult to imagine being non-harming to another. You'd never hurt babies, loved ones, neighbors, or even a stranger.

But then ask yourself how you think of others. Do you think harmful things about them? For example, "Baby is being such a pest by not letting me sleep for an hour straight! Why is she being so selfish and crying all the time to nurse? I just fed her!" or "My neighbor is so horribly inconsiderate for letting his door slam when he comes home at night. He wakes up my baby every time. He's rude and thoughtless." Consider what you say. Do you ever pick up your baby and say (even in a sweet sing-song voice), "You're being terribly annoying right now . . . did you really need to pee through another diaper after I *just* changed you? Don't you know I need to get out the door? You're being really wasteful!"

Words we say and think have power. I suggest working toward saying what we truly feel in non-harming ways. *Non-harming* invites us to discern the other side of the relationship and seek a fuller perspective on what is happening. Returning to the first example, instead of thinking that your baby is a pest for not letting you sleep, instead consider this: "Baby needs my attention a lot more often right now, and it is exhausting. I'll do my best to keep up with her needs and hope she gets through this phase soon so that I can get more sleep. It must be frustrating for her always to need another person to satisfy her needs, and it's such an honor to be the person she loves so much that I'm the one called to do it." Do you see how it is the same scenario but a complete shift in perspective and approach to satisfy the problem?

Reread the first scenario and notice how your body and mind feel when taking on the energy of harming thoughts and words. Take a breath in and out. Now read the second scenario and observe how your body and mind feel. It feels much nicer, yes? The softness you feel in your heart and body affects those around you. Once you start operating in a non-harming way, you frame your daily inter-actions with more compassion and action, not blame. This positive action initiates a chain of kindness building up your character and the actions of those around you.

Once you start operating in a non-harming way, you frame your daily interactions with more compassion and action, not blame.

You can also apply *non-harming* to how you talk, think about, and care for yourself. Do you call yourself an inadequate mother? A fail-ure? A lazy person? How is your self-image? Do you loathe parts (or all) of yourself? How can you find love and compassion for yourself in ways that motivate you to take appropriate self-care steps to nurture yourself? You may find ways to take care of yourself that are better than anyone has been able to do for you. If you tend to talk badly to yourself for eating a food you consider unhealthy, catch yourself in the moment the negative thought comes in. You have two choices: immediately think of three positive things about yourself or choose a different food that you feel is more nourishing. For example, it is 3:00 pm, and your child has refused naps any longer than twenty minutes. You are exhausted, stressed, and seek relief. You could not finish the lunch saved for yourself from last night's dinner because your child's activities pulled you away from the dining table. You reach for a handful of cookies to hold you over and instantly judge yourself, calling yourself unkind names for this choice. Stop. Think three kind things about yourself now: "I'm doing an amazing job keeping my child safe and active throughout the day," "My legs are strong and powerful, allowing me to keep up with my child," "I feel grounded through my feet as I make choices for myself and my child all day." These thoughts are rooted in actual sensations and events of the day. There is not one negative component to any of them; they all affirm your worth. Go ahead, eat the cookies without shame, and carry on with your day.

Or you can catch yourself having negative self-talk. You can observe your choice and think, "I will feel tired if I have cookies because they will not sustain me throughout this busy afternoon. I will choose carrots and peanut butter instead to feel nourished." You can go for the healthier choice and carry on. Notice that both options respect yourself. You are being kind to yourself and can act kindly towards others because you have elevated your spirit through your self-talk and actions.

TRUTHFULNESS

Truthfulness (satya) is the practice of being truthful and sincere with your thoughts, words, and actions. More than that, it's about getting real with who you are and what you want. This radical concept deserves repeating: *truthfulness* means getting real with who you are and what you want. As Deborah Adele teaches, "Real comes from the center of our unique essence and speaks to the moment from that center. Real has a boldness to it, an essence, a spontaneity. Real asks us to live from a place where there is nothing to defend and nothing to manage."[35] Living with *truthfulness* as a post for integrity means we follow through on what we feel is best for ourselves and our families. We do not agree to something for fear of hurting another's feelings. We do not overburden ourselves with tasks to project an image of Supermom who can do it all when we know fully that we will completely extinguish our inner light. Instead, *truthfulness* means tuning into your inner voice and letting it steer you to what is true and appropriate.

Do you find yourself defending your choices to yourself as if trying to convince a deeper part of yourself that your choice is correct? Or do you work at managing a lifestyle that becomes exhausting?

Truthfulness teaches that we strip away what we do not need when we get real. For example, you don't need all of the services you've hired to keep up a quality of life that may not even be an honest reflection of your real self. Suppose you pay for grocery delivery, housekeeping, satellite TV, online streaming services, a gym membership, and buy gourmet coffee drinks when you are out of the house, and you struggle to keep up with your monthly expenses. In that case, it is time to get real with what you truly need. Which of these services can you end so you can lighten your spiritual load? What if you bought your groceries and used the time choosing your meat and produce as a practice in mindfulness in which you took in the colors, sizes, textures, and smells of what looked truly good to you? You can share this practice with your child and teach the value of appreciating the colors of nature in our food. What if you made coffee at home and experimented with shaking cinnamon in the coffee grounds to make a fancy flavor? I did this as a low-income graduate student and enjoyed the flavor combinations that cost nothing to create! What if you kept either the satellite TV or the online streaming services? Do you need both? You can also ask yourself how you use the TV. Is it a distraction for your child so you can have a break? Please be honest. Can you find other activities for them so you can rest? The freedom of being honest means you do not fool yourself into being someone you are not meant to be—you do not have to be like your neighbor, best friend, or a celebrity you follow online. You can only be yourself, even if you allow yourself to stumble from time to time.

An examination of *truthfulness* begins with *you*. How consistent are your thoughts, words, and actions with one another? Do you say one thing to yourself but do something different? For example, do you say you will go to the gym three times a week and utilize the in-house childcare services only to find yourself hindered by reasons why you cannot go? Can you get real with your inconsistency? If you genuinely value fitness and feeling well, you will create opportunities to go.

Are you truthful with your expectations of what you can accomplish? If you fold in *non-harming*, are you kind to yourself when you fall short? Nicholai Bachman advises, "When [*truthfulness*] is practiced with nonviolence, the remaining *yamas* and *niyamas* become much easier."[36] Regard your energy levels throughout the day and only take on what you can realistically manage. Respect what you can do without straining yourself. It is okay to rest from time to time as well!

Are you truthful to your families and community? Do you think one thing but say or do another? If you are misaligned with how you relate to others, you will feel resentment towards them over time because you feel you must act falsely to sustain a status quo. *Truthfulness* requires a high degree of responsibility and follow-through, but it opens you to a lifestyle free from the burden and harming yourself energetically. It sets up clear intentions.

Practicing *truthfulness* affects your relationships directly. Are you in groups that support your real self? Do you allow people to be real, or do you judge, micromanage, or control others to suit your preferences? Every group has unspoken rules for what is acceptable and what creates its culture. How truthful are you to yourself when you relate to others?

As hurtful as it might feel, did your group leave you when you had your baby? What would it take from you to be real with this situation? Can you invite members of the group over to socialize and meet your baby? Of course, the social dynamics will be completely different and any expectation to do the things you used to do before the baby was born is unrealistic. If you or they believe things should be exactly as they were with the baby adding a "plus one" to the group, violates *truthfulness*. Instead, ask how the group can evolve to support you in your new phase of life. Suppose the individuals in the group cannot, then make peace with this. Trust that you will find a new group embedded in the new parenthood culture. The Community Prompts in **Part Two** will help you find others with whom you can form a group.

Any attempt on your part to act as if "life is as normal as it was before the baby" goes against the reality of your life. Everything is different with a baby. It's okay to get real with this.

Think back to the quotation from the introduction of this book that presents life occurring through seasons: "'Seasons' is a wise metaphor for the movement of life, I think...The notion that our lives are like the eternal cycle of the seasons does not deny the struggle or the joy, the loss or the gain, the darkness or the light, but encourages us to embrace it all—and to find in all of it the opportunities for growth."[37] We go through life changes from difficult to barren, vital and energetic, to sustained and content. Find what this season is for you and put forth your best, honest effort to support yourself this way while also practicing *non-harming*. What can you do that is healthful and nurturing while also nurturing your true desire?

NON-STEALING, NOT TAKING FROM OTHERS

The third *yama* is *non-stealing* (*asteya*). This guideline extends beyond the obvious action of stealing from a store or another person. Believe it or not, we steal from so many, usually in non-material ways—including from other people, the earth, and ourselves. We steal when we take more than what is given to us. If the cashier gives us back an extra dollar or charges us for conventional broccoli when we have knowingly picked organic, we are stealing if we do not say anything. Let's navigate the latter example. The farmer invested her care and energy in the organic broccoli and yielded a higher price from the store when she traded with them. The store deserves the cost of the broccoli not only because they paid more for it than the conventional but also because they have invested their environmental and social justice ethics in the farmer by supporting her work. When we point out the error in the charge, the cashier will be thankful and correct it. More importantly, you will feel energetically clearer for living with integrity (and honoring the guideline *truthfulness*).

We steal from others energetically when we limit our ability to connect with them because of jealousy, pettiness, judgment, or unkindness, especially if the other person wants to engage with you honestly. We steal others' energy when we hold back from feeling true joy for their accomplishments or find ourselves judging them to bolster ourselves. How many times have others shared the exciting news, yet you held back expressing true, unselfish joy for them because you felt envious that the same exciting thing didn't happen in your life? You may have smiled and congratulated them, but inside, you felt less excited about their experience. Coveting only takes away from your energy. What would happen if you fully walked into their joy, embraced it, and truly felt excited for them? Imagine what you'd gain energetically. By giving, you receive more.

We steal others' energy when we hold back from feeling true joy for their accomplishments or find ourselves judging them to bolster ourselves.

We steal time from others when we are late for appointments and leave scheduled meetings early. Other people value their time as much as you value yours. We live in a time where time is a currency, so let's treat it respectfully and do our best to be on time for others.

Do you show up on schedule and end sessions as planned not to steal others' time? You'll honor your schedule more when you meet others' schedules with equal respect. Do you share a balance of energy by being available for someone who needs help after this person helps you? The next time someone watches your child for an hour, allowing you to rest or run an errand, do your best to reciprocate that favor with mutual amounts of time within a reasonable timeline.

You'll honor your schedule more when you meet others' schedules with equal respect.

We steal from the earth when we take more than is needed. For example, we can be mindful not to let the water tap run while washing dishes or brushing our teeth. We can recycle items to the best of our ability and rinse them so the recycling facility can process them fast without having to discard dirty items into the landfill.

On a personal level, we steal from ourselves when we burn ourselves out doing more than we know we have to give energetically. We end up unable to listen to them, be with them, and share life experiences with them because we are too exhausted. You can be honest with how much energy you have to accomplish a task and give what's realistic. Rest when you need to restore yourself, even if it's only ten minutes.

You steal from yourself when you let anxiety get the best of you and stay focused on future "what ifs." Anxiety lives in an imagined future. There is no truth to the anxious thoughts because they live in fantasy and not in what is happening now. Feel your breath, get grounded, and live in the moment. Be honest with what is happening in front of you. Realize the life you want to have and stay grounded to create that moment piece by piece. You can write out your vision for your life that illustrates how you feel when you have a balance of energy and freedom in your work, relationships, hobbies and passions, self-care, and finances. Set up a savings account to invest in what is important to you. Can you set aside even five percent of your monthly income and use those funds for a massage every so often? Invest in the relationships that are most important to you—the *real* you—and let go of toxic ones that bring you down. Anyone who steals energy from you is not worth your concern. Can you find a kind and honest way to preserve your energy and protect yourself from their toxicity?

Remember, the opposite of stealing is investing—invest in yourself, invest in others, and invest in sustaining the environment your child will inherit from you.

Remember, the opposite of stealing is investing—invest in yourself, invest in others, and invest in sustaining the environment your child will inherit from you.

NON-EXCESS, THE CONSERVATION OF VITAL ENERGY

The fourth guideline is *non-excess*, also known as *conservation of vital energy (brahmacharya)*. This lesson teaches us to send our energy in positive directions rather than focus on an excess of substances, sex, shopping, or other vices. Placing too much energy into vices robs us of energy we could use to clarify our spiritual life and capacity to connect fully with others. *Non-excess* teaches us to cherish the material possessions we believe are essential and let go of the rest. Why buy lots of plastic storage bins to stash away objects if you only forget what is in the bins over time? How would it feel if you cleared them out, donated what was usable for others, and freed up your living and energetic spaces?

This does not mean you keep only the dishes you use in a day and live sparsely. It means getting real about what's truly important to you. For example, because I wouldn't say I like dusting, I no longer have small decorative items and small picture frames lining shelves. I find it tedious to dust all of them! Moreover, freeing up this clutter opens my living space and allows me to feel more relaxed in my home so I can tend to what's important to me.

We might also take more than we need, especially with food. In an extreme yet realistic example, consider the all-you-can-eat buffets. I noticed myself being excessive at East Indian lunch buffets, eating two (sometimes three) full plates of food! I had to ask myself, "When do I ever eat two or three plates of food in my normal life? I don't! Then why do I need more, just because I'm at this buffet?" I'd walk away feeling stuffed, bloated, and riddled with indigestion that lasted the rest of the day. But I've learned to manage my plate appropriately and only use a second plate for cold items such as green salad or chutneys. This new behavior was an act of kindness for myself, an honest expression of what I truly needed, and did not take more than I needed from the restaurant or the others in the buffet line. You can see how the other *yamas* relate to one another when you live ethically.

In your life, do you eat when you feel you've been satisfied by what was on your plate? Or do you keep eating because it tastes good, or do you believe you must clean your plate? The next time you overeat, notice how the food tastes, and ask if it tastes as good as your first hungry bite. Chances are, you'd say the food isn't as flavorful. Your body has an intelligent way of preserving optimal digestion by dulling the taste buds once satiation occurs. Do honor this body wisdom. It is a tool for non-excess to preserve your vital energy.

Your body has an intelligent way of preserving optimal digestion by dulling the taste buds once satiation occurs. Do honor this body wisdom.

Indeed, we tend to also fall into addictions of many types. From coffee to TV shows to controlled substances to sex and physical affection, our habits tend to manage us and rob us of energy to do the Divine work we are meant to do in our lifetime. What would happen if, after wanting one more cup of coffee, for example, you instead drank a small glass of water, sat still, and just breathed, eyes closed? Do this and notice the sensation of what you need, and then tend to that. If you are tired, rest for five minutes or so. If you are thirsty, drink more water. If you notice you are lonely and feeding an emptiness inside, call someone you care about to say hello.

The more real we get with what we truly need to live dynamically, the more we can tend to our inner selves and the Divine around us. As a mother, how can you conserve your vital energy to best do the work that uplifts and honors your spirit? Once you distill your vital resources into what is truly important, you can have a freer exchange of energy with others while taking care of yourself.

NON-HOARDING

The fifth *yama* is *non-hoarding* (*aparigraha*). We may initially think of the TV programs that reveal the intense clutter in people's homes. This is an extreme example of hoarding. On subtler levels, hoarding happens when we grip too tightly onto objects, people, our bodies, or our thoughts. We tend to grasp firmly onto objects and not want to release our hold on items, *even if we no longer use them as we once did.*

Have you kept the jeans you bought years ago, holding out for the day you'll wear them again? How much energy is that draining from you? How would it feel to let go of the jeans and the idea of who you feel you would be if you wore them? What could you manifest with the newfound energy you have? Are you holding onto objects from yesteryear that represented a person you used to be with hopes you are still the same? We constantly evolve and often outgrow things that no longer meet the needs of our current life. This concept of impermanence teaches us that nothing stays the same day to day. It is futile and robs our energy to clutch to what was. Instead, find contentment with what is *right now*. When we release our attachment to things, we free our energy to care for ourselves and our families better.

When we release our attachment to things, we free our energy to care for ourselves and our families better.

We also practice this lesson by not holding rigid opinions or controlling others. What would happen if you let people surprise you instead of judging them against an idea of who they are? For instance, what if you support someone taking up an exercise regimen instead of labeling him as "the lazy one" and expecting him to fail? Can you genuinely support him in his actions and feel true joy at his successes?

Part of the practice of *non-hoarding* of rigid opinions is to allow others to speak and act freely. Be present with your neighbors if they discuss their beliefs about an issue instead of shutting out any idea different from your own. On a more intimate level, be open-hearted about who your child is. Do you label your child and hold onto an opinion about them? Do you label them a "bad sleeper" if they have trouble sleeping? Notice how this binds your energy around the entire topic and practice of sleeping. Instead, soften your heart to the idea that your child has a challenge, and you are working toward solving it. Every day, affirm a genuine love and support for yourself, knowing you and your baby will figure it out. Be open to new approaches to sleeping; be kind to yourself and your child as you navigate this particular path.

Every day, affirm a genuine love and support for yourself, knowing you and your child will figure it out.

What thoughts do you hold onto about yourself? Do you continually call yourself lazy, messy, or some other condescending label? Do you keep yourself in a cage as you grab onto unkind or false ideas about your capabilities? Instead, stay rooted in the present moment. Be honest with your energy, tap into the Divine light within, and act according to your genuine needs that serve your real self. Don't nurture the possible inauthentic self you may project to satisfy an imagined standard. If you are still trapped in inauthenticity, revisit *truthfulness*.

The Niyamas: Loving Yourself

While the *yamas* provide ethical guidelines for being in a relationship with the world, the *niyamas* teach us how to create and nurture our best selves.

Niyama translates to "internal control or restraint."[38] Through a series of disciplined practices, we distill out any unnecessary actions that dampen our inner light and prevent us from honoring our pure selves. This is the time to take care of ourselves profoundly and spiritually.

CLEANLINESS, PURITY

The first *niyama* is *cleanliness and purity (śaucha)*. This personal practice helps us maintain a clean body and clear heart-mind. We clear ourselves of toxins emotionally, mentally, and physically to better receive others. On a daily level, we bathe regularly, eat whole foods that are as organic as we can afford, and move often. Good hygiene leaves of feeling fresh and balanced. Clean eating energizes and purifies the body from within. Moving daily in various ways flushes the lymphatic system, helps the heart pump blood efficiently throughout the body, and keeps the channels open. Notice the correlation between clearing your body and how it affects the clarity of your mind.

Notice the correlation between clearing your body and how it affects the clarity of your mind.

Chances are, once you eat more cleanly and detoxify your body, you will be more balanced in your emotions, and your thoughts will be kinder and more balanced. Deborah Adele teaches, "Cleansing strengthens the body and insulates the mind, preparing us for the awakening of energy within us. Cleansing prepares us for the greatness of our spirit."[39]

Start by drinking more water, eating more vegetables (the greener and leafier, the better), and adding more walks to your daily routine. Notice what new energy comes up. Consciously speak in kind ways to purify your thoughts and words. Give thanks often and notice the change in your heart. Sometimes you might "come clean" by admitting a fault and releasing a deeply held emotion. How can you peel back the layers of *cleanliness* to reveal a balanced and clear self?

The practice of *cleanliness* also relates to the places we inhabit. We work toward uncluttering our surroundings to focus our energies inward to an uncluttered heart. Notice how clutter and heavy piles of objects weigh down your spirit. How would it feel to release that clutter and free up your inner space and surroundings? What could you accomplish in your daily life if you had room to move, breathe, and live fully in your surroundings?

Sometimes a cluttered home mirrors a cluttered heart-mind. Does this ring true for you? As you look at the amount of "stuff" in your home, question what you truly need. Describe how your sense of self is reflected in your home and surroundings. Please start with the outer environment and notice how it affects you inwardly when you organize and clean your spaces. Or get real on what things you need. Even better, create a vision for how you want your space to reflect you and your core values.

Get real on what things you need. Even better, create a vision for how you want your space to reflect you and your core values.

Of course, babies and children have "stuff." Is there a way to manage your belongings so they don't take over? Can you donate or sell toys your child has developmentally outgrown? Can you do the same with clothing and books? What about sippy cups and utensils your child no longer needs to use? All these questions incorporate *non-hoarding.*

The more you release, the clearer you will find the energy moving in your home. You may be surprised at how your relationships with your family improve when you release clutter and purify the spaces you share with them. This contributes to creating a home that reflects the purity you create in your body, mind, and spirit. The more you meet the actual needs of yourself and your child by releasing outdated objects and supporting yourself and them with tools appropriate for their stage of life, the more you can embrace what's happening and continue forward with your child as you grow on this path together.

The practice of *cleanliness* means we get real and present with what is happening in ourselves and around us. We receive those happenings with pure thoughts, words, and actions. The more we move through life as an act of mindfulness free from judgment, the more we release violence from our heart-mind and find purity within. This cleans our spirit and helps us shine forth truly and authentically.

The more we move through life as an act of mindfulness free from judgment, the more we release violence from our

heart-mind and find purity within. This cleans our spirit and helps us shine forth truly and authentically.

CONTENTMENT AND GRATITUDE

The second *niyama* is *contentment and gratitude* (*santosha*). In this practice, we work toward expressing gratitude for what we have, for who we are, and for where we are in life. We work against the tendency common in human nature to strive for something more extravagant than what we have. Release the idea that there's something better for you than you already possess—work against feeling envious of what others have and downplaying what you have in your life. Instead, find the beauty in appreciating what you have, your relationships, and who you are.

Can you feel content, balanced, and pleased with who you are and what you've accomplished without striving for something different? Can you feel satisfied with what is in your life? Feel gratitude for what you have and be content with where you are.

Feel gratitude for what you have and be content with where you are.

This is not to say you don't set goals for your personal growth—an important part of personal and professional development. The difference lies in how you receive your path. Can you feel content with every step, each action, and even every setback as you find your path taking you toward your vision for yourself?

Contentment is directly related to being unattached to the results of your actions. If you work toward a goal and the result is less than what you expected, instead of being disappointed or angry, accept what happens, learn from it, and move on with your life. Even better and more in alignment with *contentment*, be satisfied with the lessons you gained from the process. In this way, you cultivate gratitude without finding the need to seek more. Deborah Adele teaches, "Practicing *gratitude* protects us from our pettiness and smallness and keeps us centered in the joy and abundance of our own life."[40]

Gratitude nourishes our heart-mind and creates a sense of fulfillment. It is truly the practice of being present. We feel content with what we have and what we learn in every waking moment. This is true, even if our circumstances aren't great, such as dealing with an illness or losing finances. In these moments, can we still feel content with the lessons we learn or with what we still have? Every setback is an opportunity to learn about your choices and set you on a new path to something better. Can you find *gratitude* in the lessons?

As a mother, you strive to be content with the energy you have put forth taking care of yourself, your child, and your family. Don't compare yourself to other mothers; be content with your own path and process. You are exactly where you need to be at this moment in time. You are in the process of self-betterment and spiritual clarity that is opening you continuously to your path to your best self.

As a mother, you strive to be content with the energy you have put forth taking care of yourself, your child, and your family.

PRACTICE CAUSING POSITIVE CHANGE

The third *niyama* is creating a *practice causing deliberate change* (*tapas*). We often feel stuck in habits and patterns that sabotage our wellness efforts. For example, you may start an exercise regimen to gain more energy and lose a bit of holiday weight gain. Even though you feel motivated at the beginning, old thought patterns creep in, saying you cannot follow through in this new endeavor. You tell yourself that the time you created for jogging is time you should use for your job or cleaning the house. You may feel guilty and stop exercising, which puts you right back where you started—feeling stuck!

You can create an intention for *practice causing deliberate change* and can deliberately act in a way that causes a positive change in our lives.[41] Your intention is your dedication to yourself that you honor and build upon every time you follow through on your vision for self-betterment. Creating discipline heats mental, physical, and emotional impurities that keep you feeling stuck energetically. Like how fire (with effort) can transform steel into a sharp sword, the heat you create transforms you into a higher self.

When we consciously change a habit that holds us back, discomfort arises and creates friction in the bodymind. We learn to be comfortable with discomfort through a daily practice of self-awareness and then choose the action we intuitively know is healthful for us. As Deborah Adele writes, "[*Practice causing deliberate change*] is the day-to-day choice to burn non-supportive habits of the body and mind, choosing to forsake momentary pleasures for future rewards."[42]

We initiate *practice causing deliberate change* by dedicating ourselves to a daily yoga practice in which we determine what's safe for us and what we can explore further. Ask these questions:

- What is the best effort you can put into your practice?
- Where do you need to back off and include more restorative poses or rest?
- How can you be more disciplined with nutrition and eat primarily foods that nourish the body?

Remember to be kind to yourself and discover the balance between discipline and deprivation. When you find yourself pulled towards old habits that keep you stuck, make it an invitation to dive inwardly. What grips you? Breathe into it. When you create a discipline that fosters a pure self, your higher self awaits on the other side.

When you create a discipline that fosters a pure self, your higher self awaits on the other side.

Your *practice of causing deliberate change* comes with much discomfort because it's hard to break debilitating habits and adopt healthful habits. You might get an immediate rush when you start a new practice and see results after a week—a boost in energy or a loss of a pound or two. But what happens in Week Four when you reach a plateau or things get tough and desperately want to return to your old ways? This is when the heat turns up. Find your focus, feel your breath, and stay the course.

The transformation from *practice causing deliberate change* occurs when you consciously practice day after day. You come into your practice every time you step onto your mat (or into your kitchen if your goal is more healthful eating). You resolve to put forth your best effort of what's available for you energetically that day. Please do your best with what you have and sit with any discomfort as it arises. Deborah Adele writes, "[*Practice causing deliberate change*] is growing our ability to stay in the unknown and the unpleasantness, rather than run in fear."[43] In doing so, you gain so much and shed what doesn't serve you.

What habits do you have that hold you back or prevent you from being well? Whether you feel constrained by poor nutrition, a lack of movement that results in energy stagnation, or any other lack of energy that disconnects you from your spiritual life, begin your practice with courage. Then you can stand in the fire of the discipline and work toward transforming your physical, mental, and spiritual self.

Begin your practice with courage so you can stand in the fire of discipline.

STUDY BY AND OF ONESELF

The fourth niyama is the *study by and of oneself* (svādhyāya). This guideline for self-love is about developing one's heart-mind by recognizing the layers of our ego/identity and peeling them away to get to our radiant being within. This starts and ends with studying yourself from within.

Like the Russian nesting (matryoshka) dolls, our sense of self has many layers and identities. We have who we are in public, who we are to our parents, who we are to our partners, who we are to our children, etc. The layers run deep. We work through *the practices causing deliberate change* and *self-study* to observe ourselves in action and get to the core of who we are. It is natural to have variance between you at work and home. However, if you feel spiritual discord because of misalignments in how you show up in the world to different people, I invite you to spend more time in meditation to explore this.

Deep within, we find Divinity at our center. Some may identify it as God; others may call it Universal Nature. Whatever name you give it, it's always there from birth and with you. Untainted, it's your true nature. This essential self does not need healing—it is pure. The layers that surround it are either mutable or fixed; in this case, they become boxes that cage us in. Deborah Adele says, "Self-study is about knowing our true identity as Divine and understanding the boxes we are wrapped in. We can find clues about our boxes by watching our projections, by the process of tracing our reactions back to a belief, and by courageously looking at life as it is."44

We live in a layered self to function in the world. The work of yoga is to bring awareness to our strengths and shortcomings through meditation, *asana* practice, breath-centered awareness, and reading/listening/learning that promote self-reflection and insightful observation of ourselves in action. Once we understand where we are on our path, we can set an intention to let go of our negative qualities (through *practice causing deliberate change*) and reinforce the attributes that positively affect ourselves and others.

Nicholai Bachman shares, "*Practice causing change* naturally leads to *self-study* as we observe the changes happening and adjust our practice to maintain our desired direction. It may be easier to wait until the heat diminishes, then in a quieter space, reflect on the *practice causing change* experience."[45] You will find over time how the different ways to relate to various groups in your life become more and more the same. In short, you may realize how you have softened your skin and become more of who you truly are to all people. You find your agency as yourself and stand firmly in that light.

Please keep up a meditation practice as you navigate these final three niyamas so you can see how these principles are in daily life.

In the postnatal stage of life, *self-study* comes when we consciously choose to learn about ourselves while inhabiting the role of Mother. Every instructional or philosophical book you read on taking care of your child is an opportunity to find *your* values shaping how you care for yourself and your family. All actions and interactions are moments for learning. You can use this time to know who you truly are and make changes to let go of any actions, thoughts, and attitudes that do not serve you.

You can use this time to come to know who you truly are and make changes to let go of any actions, thoughts, and attitudes that do not serve you.

In addition, notice your reactions to what life brings you. Deborah Adele teaches, "Every event that life presents to us is a precious opportunity to learn the truth about the boxes we have ourselves packaged in."[46] If you observe and choose to learn from events, notice if you think of yourself as a victim when unfortunate things happen. Or can you have a sense of humor about how crazy life can be? Your perspective on life determines how you position yourself in the world. Find ways to take responsibility for your choices when an event happens because of the work you have put out in the world. If you are involved in a tragic event or a loss, can you find kindness for yourself without blaming yourself?

Even when you are exhausted, you can always feel your breath and draw your awareness inward to notice how you react and live with the circumstances in your life. If you find strife, what can you do to find peace? Can you adopt a new perspective to shift from *reactive* to *proactive* when life gives you lemons? How do you make lemonade that benefits the situation and helps you discover something about yourself? Can you find compassion for yourself along the way, knowing that to be human is to be imperfect? And it is much better to be true to yourself imperfectly than live a lie as somebody else perfectly. You can only be you. Find peace with the brilliance you bring to the world.

Can you find compassion for yourself along the way, knowing that to be human is to be imperfect?

SURRENDER TO THE DIVINE

The tenth principle and last of the *niyamas* is *surrendering to the Divine*, which comes with the ebb and flow of life to connect with God's will.

We find humility when we do this. We don't have to meditate for two hours to feel this principle in action. If you have explored the five *yamas* and the four *niyamas* thus far, you may have already experienced the freedom of surrender. You have found ways to truly relate with other people and receive them as they are while being content with what you bring.

When you gaze into your child's eyes, and they lovingly look back at you, you *surrender to the divine*. It's an undeniable presence of Divinity between the two of you. You are content, pure inside, and grateful for what you have. You surrender to any imagined shortcomings you have, and you're fully absorbed—you're one with the moment.

The heart of this *niyama* presupposes a Divine force at work in our lives.[47] We tap into the Divine nature within us through meditation, prayer, and the healing art of yoga. We create *practice causing change* to transform ourselves into our best selves and use much *self-study* to get to what is real.

At the center of it all is Divinity. It is both within and surrounding us all the time. Moreover, it is there for us when we need it—all we have to do is breathe and find our grounding to access it. Deborah Adele teaches, "This guideline invites us to surrender our egos, open our hearts and accept the higher purpose of our being."[48]

Surrender to the Divine does not mean giving up and letting go of integrity. Instead, it means finding your inner-felt resources and using them to navigate your path, knowing the Divine deeply cares about you and supports you along the way. You have the tools you need to explore your life. Moreover, you are creating more tools throughout *The Postpartum Path of Yoga* program. Be kind to yourself. Listen to your inner voice and trust your intuition. By heeding this, you can soften your skin and let go when you need to trust in the Higher Power. You cannot white-knuckle your way through life and feel freedom. Instead, find the balance between effort and relaxation in your daily life, just as you do in your mindful movement practice.

You cannot white-knuckle your way through life and feel freedom. Instead, you find the balance between effort and relaxation in your daily life, just as you do in your mindful movement practice.

If we go too hard and rigid through life, we miss out on all of the feelings and sensations waiting for us if we could have accepted them with more vulnerability. *Surrender to the Divine* invites us to go with the flow, ride out the waves, and enjoy the freedom of not planning everything along the way. As John Lennon sang in *Beautiful Boy*, "Life is what happens while you're busy making other plans." Don't miss out on your life. We can open our eyes, ears, and heart to what's happening from moment to moment and enjoy it as it comes.

Final Questions for Reflection

In **Part Four**, you have observed your thoughts, words, and actions in daily life. Now consider these questions:

- Have you found that you live through a principle of *non-harming*?
- Are you *honest* with who you are as you present yourself to others? Are you *real* with yourself as you define your needs?
- Do you *take only what you need* and no more?
- Do you *conserve your resources* (food, energy, finances, sensory experiences, sexual energy) so you can live without excess and waste? How can you manifest a higher purpose if you practice moderation with these resources?
- Do you grasp onto material possessions, or can you *freely let go* of items that no longer serve your life? Do you clutch onto an idea of what your life is "supposed" to be instead of being open to where things are right now?
- How much energy do you put into *cleanliness* for yourself (nutrition, exercise, hygiene) and your home? Are you over-zealous with cleanliness in a way that is obsessive (which is harmful)? Do you take care of yourself well?
- Are you *grateful* for what you have and do not feel jealous over what others have? What makes you feel *content* in your life? How much is "just enough"?
- What *practices* can you do that will cause you to dismantle unhealthy habits so you can *cultivate your pure self*? What habits do you need to release to clarify your inner-felt spirit? What can you do to inspire this transformation?

- Are you observing and *studying yourself* at the moment without judgment? What are you learning about yourself as a layered and dynamic being? Are you behaving in inauthentic ways? Or are you honoring your true self?
- Are you *connected to a Divine source* larger than yourself that humbles you? Do you have faith that this source is always inside and around you and deeply cares for you?
- Can you find this Divinity in other people as you serve family and community? How can you fully let go of your ego to submit yourself to a higher force and find true bliss?

The *yamas* and *niyamas* are codes and guidelines that live with you your whole life. As you move from one season and phase of life to another, take time to dive into these practices as a course of study. You want to live through them as a template for daily ethical life. The more you strip away what isn't necessary now, the better you can go with the flow and enjoy moments as they come. Bliss lies within; it's ready for you.

Take care of yourself and those around you, and you will inhabit it again and again.

~ 6 ~

CLOSING REMARKS

You have been through a journey throughout *The Postpartum Path of Yoga* program. You have adopted practices that open your heart-mind and allow you to examine yourself. If you have tended to these practices regularly, you have noticed a shift in how you feel physically, emotionally, and perhaps spiritually. You have created fertile grounds for your growth and development as a woman and mother. B.K.S. Iyengar, the famed teacher of modern yoga, equates a life framed by yoga as a tree in his book *The Tree of Yoga*. When you embrace the eight limbs of a yoga practice—the *yamas*, *niyamas*, *asana* (the poses), *pranayama* (breath control), *pratyahara* (sensory withdrawal to immerse inwardly in oneself), *dharana* (concentration), *dhyana* (meditation), and *samadhi* (bliss), you find the tree's limbs support you and your life flourishes beautifully. I will elaborate on his metaphor in hopes that you recall your experiences through *The Postpartum Path of Yoga* program so you can embody these more extensive teachings.

Iyengar describes the influence of the eight limbs on one's life as the parts of a tree. The *yamas* create the tree's roots because they ground the practitioner as she works toward discerning her perceptions and her mind. The *yamas* anchor her principles and prepare her for what's to come in life. You have discovered that the yamas clarified your ethics and principles as you reflected upon and enacted them daily.

The *niyamas* create the trunk of the tree because they make up how the practitioner relates to herself and the world more fully through her senses. You feel more solid and connected to your core self through studying the *niyamas*. From the trunk emerge several branches that move in different directions—some twisted, some straight, some curved. These branches are the *asanas* that move the body in different orientations as the practitioner strives to find inner harmony through them. You may have expanded your self-awareness as you moved in many ways in poses like *Staff Pose*, *Gate Pose*, and *Marichi's Pose C*.

From the branches grow leaves that interact with the air. Leaves take in carbon dioxide, release oxygen, and capture the sunshine to create food for the tree through photosynthesis. The leaves represent *pranayama*, or breathing practices that rejuvenate and sustain the body and mind. The tree branches are covered with bark that protects the tree and preserves its inward flow of energy. The bark represents *pratyahara*, or the sensorial path inward to investigate oneself. You discovered the importance of sustaining an inward focus as you experienced the subtle and overt power of the breath-based practices in this program.

The tree's sap is *dharana*, or concentration because it feeds the mind's capacity to connect with the body and the spirit. The ability to concentrate on sensation and the bodymind-in-action nourishes your mind. The tree's sap moves from the core of one's being to the tip of the roots—from deep within to the periphery. This represents *dhyana*, or meditation. You may have discovered how essential concentration is to your meditation practice and how effortlessly you can create it over time. Meditation practice makes the flowers on the tree. Finally, when the flower blossoms into fruit, this is *samadhi*, or bliss, representing the connection to the Divine within and all around.[49] You may have tapped into this bliss early on, or it may have manifested later. Once you feel it and know its pathway, isn't it a relief to know how to come into bliss through this range of yoga practices? Realize you have the personal power and freedom to get there to support your spirit and nurture your personal development.

Now that you have completed this program, you may relate to Iyengar's metaphor of the tree. You may sense how your created practices and disciplines can ground and liberate you at once. I love trees. Trees anchor themselves, expand through the air, sustain life, and communicate with other trees through their root systems. They are truly remarkable organisms. Although they look fixed on the outside, they can steadily adapt to changes in their environment. You can find your grounding, grow, adapt, and grow in many seasons of motherhood.

You can find your grounding, grow, adapt, and grow in the many seasons of motherhood.

The yogic guidelines and the physiological and anatomical lessons in **Part One** teach you the groundwork for laying your soil. Regard them as the circumstances of your environment now, but they are changeable, and you can grow beyond them. They never limit you.

The practices in **Part Two** and **Part Three** provide resources to branch out, explore new possibilities, tap into the potent-yet-subtle power of your breath, and tune inwards. You do this through active meditation, mindful movement, connected vocal expression, and finding stillness within seated meditation. Your work in **Part Four** with the *yamas* and *niyamas* deepens your roots and further refines your spiritual growth and personal refinement. You tune into the deep-felt integrity and ethics that uplift you every day. You feel the sap lying dormant inside you while it nurtures your spirit and connects you to the Divine.

Your work may start peripherally with the physical body but moves deep within. You discover the point at which your effort radiates back out. That's when you feel connected, whole, and committed to your self-care and spiritual growth. Moreover, you can navigate this program repeatedly and always find something new. With each season of life, feel your breath, and come onto your yoga mat. Attune with yourself and look within.

With each season of life, feel your breath, and come onto your yoga mat. Attune with yourself and look within.

The work begins whenever you intend to adapt to life's changes and surrender to the possibilities. I wish you all the best in your restoration, wellness, and self-love path.

ABOUT THE AUTHOR

Melissa Hurt is a certified yoga teacher (700 hrs), a Lessac Certified Trainer of Kinesensic voice, speech, and movement, and the owner of Integrative Studio, LLC in Delmar, New York.

For more than a decade, Melissa has shared embodiment practices across the United States and in Sydney, Australia, at universities, yoga studios, and yoga teacher trainings. She incorporates breath-centered practices, mindful movement, embodied voice practices, and meditation in her classes to bring students to embodied wholeness in body, mind, voice, and spirit. They turn to their inner-felt resources to care for themselves and live with vitality, balance, and loving-kindness.

Melissa has a Ph.D. in Theatre Arts (concentration in actor training) from the University of Oregon and an MFA in Theatre Pedagogy from Virginia Commonwealth University. She integrates her knowledge of performance training, the actor's process, theatre production, and embodiment practices in her corporate coaching.

Melissa is the author of I Am the Jungle: A Yoga Adventure (Sounds True Publishing 2020), Arthur Lessac's Embodied Actor Training (Routledge 2014), and several articles for Voice and Speech Review, Theatre Topics, Theatre Symposium, Collective Writings on the Lessac Voice and Body Work (Llumina Press 2010), and a chapter on mindfulness practice in Play with Purpose: Lessac Kinesensics in Action (LTRI 2017).

You can learn more about Melissa and her online offerings at www.melissahurt.com. Deepen your personal development with the teachings on her YouTube channel: www.youtube.com/c/MelissaHurt.

ACKNOWLEDGEMENTS

I would not be who I am today as a woman or as an embodiment teacher without many people's love, support, and guidance.

I am thankful for all my yoga and meditation teachers over my years of practice. A few hold a deep seat in my heart: Vandana (my first yoga teacher who taught with grace, knowledge, and compassion), Simon Borg-Olivier (a teacher who taught me the most about intelligent practice and the importance of living yoga in daily life), Bianca Machliss (a teacher who answered my questions honestly and compassionately as I practiced while pregnant and postnatally), and Lori Ritland (who shares a deep reverence for the Iyengar practice and modified practices to heal my postnatal body). I am grateful for my yoga family at Sun and Moon Yoga Studio.

I am thankful for the practitioners and certified trainers of the Lessac Training and Research Institute®, particularly Deb Kinghorn and Nancy Krebs. I am indebted to their ongoing guidance, support, and friendship. I thank Arthur Lessac for the support and teaching he gave me for years before his passing. His voice guides me along my path whenever I share embodied voice practices.

I am thankful for my family and friends who have believed in me and supported my work as an embodiment coach. Thank you for holding space for what I do and never asking me to change who I am.

I am deeply grateful for the support and love of my daughter, Penny. I could not do what I do without her as the foundation of my life.

I can only fulfill my dharma as a teacher if I have someone to teach. I am deeply grateful for every student I have ever taught embodiment practices. Thank you for showing up, asking questions, digging deep, and doing the work. Your growth inspires me, and I vow to continue helping as many people as possible.

I thank God for giving me the courage, grace, and humility to realize my shortcomings and the wisdom to open my eyes and find the tools I need to evolve.

BIBLIOGRAPHY

Adele, Deborah. *The Yamas and Niyamas: Exploring Yoga's Ethical Practice.* Duluth, MN: On-Word Bound Books LLC, 2009.

Bachman, Nicholai. *The Yoga Sutras Workbook.* Boulder, Colorado: Sounds True Publishing, 2010.

Blum, Haley. "Totally Fried." *The ASHA Leader,* February 2016, Vol. 21, 50-56. https://leader.pubs.asha.org/article.aspx?articleid=2485708

Bowman, Katy. *Diastasis Recti: The Whole-Body Solution to Abdominal Weakness and Separation.* USA: Propriometrics Press, 2016.

Cacioppo, John T. & William Patrick. *Loneliness: Human Nature and the Need for Social Connection.* New York, NY: W.W. Norton & Company, 2008.

Calais-Germain, Blandine. *The Female Pelvis: Anatomy & Exercises.* Seattle, WA: Eastland Press, Inc., 2003.

Feuerstein, Georg. Trans. *The Bhagavad-Gita: A New Translation.* Boston, MA : Shambhala Publications, Inc., 2011.

Hanson, Rick. *Buddha's Brain: The Practical Neuroscience of Happiness, Love, & Wisdom.* California: New Harbinger Publications, Inc., 2014.

Iyengar, B.K.S. *Light on Life: The Yoga Journey to Wholeness, Inner Peace, and Ultimate*

--- ---. *The Tree of Yoga.* Boston: Shambhala Publications, Inc, 1988.

Kempton, Sally. *Meditation for the Love of It: Enjoying Your Own Deepest Experience.* Boulder, Colorado: Sounds True Publishing, 2011.

Lennon, John. "Beautiful Boy" from the *Double Fantasy* album. 1980.

Lessac, Arthur. *The Use and Training of the Human Voice: A Bio-Dynamic Approach to Vocal Life*, 3rd edition. USA: McGraw-Hill, 1996.

Lessac, Arthur and Deborah Kinghorn. *Essential Lessac: Honoring the Familiar in Body, Mind, Spirit.* NH: RMJ Donald Publishing, 2014.

Lieberman, Matthew D. *Social: Why Our Brains Are Wired to Connect.* New York: Crown Publishers, 2013.

Madill, Cate. "Keep An Eye On Vocal Fry." https://theconversation.com/keep-an-eye-on-vocal-fry-its-all-about-power-status-and-gender-45883. July 1, 2018.

Mercado, Jocelyn. "Send Peace and Happiness Into the World: Loving Kindness Meditation. https://blog.pachamama.org/send-peace-and-happiness-into-the-world-loving-kindness-meditation.   June 20, 2015.

McCulloch Dip, Sam. "Postnatal Depletion: What It Is and How To Recover." https://www.bellybelly.com.au/post-natal/postnatal-depletion-what-it-is-and-how-to-recover/ October 2017.

Nicks, Stevie. "Landslide" from the *Fleetwood Mac* album. 1975.

Palmer, Parker J. *Let Your Life Speak: Listening for the Voice of Vocation.* San Francisco, CA: Jossey-Bass, 1999.

Serrallach, Oscar. *The Postnatal Depletion Cure: A Complete Guide to Rebuilding Your Health and Reclaiming Your Energy for Mothers of Newborns, Toddlers, and Young Children.* New York, NY: Hachette Book Group, 2018.

Starr, Rebecca Fox. *Beyond the Baby Blues: Anxiety and Depression During and After Pregnancy.* MD: Rowman & Littlefield Publishers, 2017.

Zimmer, Carl. "In a Mother's Milk, Nutrients and a Message, Too." *NY Times* November 16, 2014. https://www.nytimes.com/2014/11/06/science/in-a-mothers-milk-nutrients-and-a-message-too.html

ENDNOTES

[1] Parker Palmer J. *Let Your Life Speak: Listening for the Voice of Vocation.* (Jossey-Bass, 1999), p. 46.

[2] Stevie Nicks sang this answer to her question in her live performance in a performance published online by American Express on March 3, 2010.

[3] *Let Your Life Speak* (Jossey-Bass, 1999). p. 102.

[4] Translated by Nicolai Bachman from *The Yoga Sutras Workbook.* (Sounds True, 2010).

[5] Arthur Lessac is a famed originator of a voice, speech, and movement modality popularly used in actor training programs around the world. His work has also been used by corporate professionals, healthcare professionals, lawyers, and anyone interested in developing a dynamic speaking voice as felt from within via the tono-sensory process. His most popular book, *The Use and Training of the Human Voice*, was first published in 1963. It's in its third edition, published by McGraw-Hill in 1996.

[6] Iyengar, B.K.S. *The Tree of Yoga,* Boston, MA: Shambhala Classics, 2002. pp. 46-47

[7] McCulloch Dip, Sam. "Postnatal Depletion: What It Is and How To Recover." https://www.bellybelly.com.au/post-natal/postnatal-depletion-what-it-is-and-how-to-recover/ October 2017.

[8] Serrallach, Oscar. *The Postnatal Depletion Cure: A Complete Guide to Rebuilding Your Health and Reclaiming Your Energy for Mothers of Newborns, Toddlers, and Young Children.* (Hachette Book Group, 2018), p. 5.

[9] McCulloch Dip, Sam. "Postnatal Depletion: What It Is and How To Recover." https://www.bellybelly.com.au/post-natal/post-natal-depletion-what-it-is-and-how-to-recover/ October 2017.

[10] Zimmer, Carl. "In a Mother's Milk, Nutrients and a Message, Too." NY Times November 16, 2014. https://www.nytimes.com/2014/11/06/science/in-a-mothers-milk-nutrients-and-a-message-too.html

[11] Lieberman, Matthew D. *Social: Why Our Brains Are Wired to Connect.* (Crown Publishers, 2013), p. 43.

[12] Starr, Rebecca Fox. *Beyond the Baby Blues: Anxiety and Depression During and After Pregnancy* (Rowman & Littlefield Publishers, 2017), p. 92.

[13] Madill, Cate. "Keep An Eye On Vocal Fry." https://theconversation.com/keep-an-eye-on-vocal-fry-its-all-about-power-status-and-gender-45883. July 1, 2018.

[14] Blum, Haley. "Totally Fried." *The ASHA Leader*, February 2016, Vol. 21, pp. 50-56. https://leader.pubs.asha.org/article.aspx?articleid=2485708

[15] Arthur Lessac and Deborah Kinghorn. *Essential Lessac: Honoring the Familiar in Body, Mind, Spirit.* (RMJ Donald Publishing, 2014), p. 124.

[16] *The Tree of Yoga.* (Shambhala Classics, 2002) p. 42.

[17] Learn more about Iyengar's description of concentration and meditation in *The Tree of Yoga* (Shambhala Classics, 2002) pp. 41-43.

[18] Fitzpatrick, Lisa. "The Vagus Nerve: Secrets to a Sustainable Nervous System." Presentation from L1 Restorative Yoga Teacher Training: Module "Understanding the Vagus Nerve in More Depth," Bliss Baby Yoga. 2018.

[19] Hanson, Rick. *Buddha's Brain: The Practical Neuroscience of Happiness, Love, & Wisdom.* (New Harbinger Publications, Inc.: 2014) p. 42.

[20] Ibid. pp. 68-69.

[21] To read more about Arthur Lessac's description of the reverse megaphone, see *The Use and Training of the Human Voice*, 3rd edition (McGraw-Hill ,1996), pp. 161-164.

[22] Blandine Calais-Germain. *The Female Pelvis: Anatomy & Exercises*. (Eastland Press, Inc., 2003), pp. 112-113.

[23] Ibid. (Eastland Press, Inc., 2003) pp.108-114.

[24] See Katy Bowman's *Diastasis Recti* (Propriometrics Press, 2016) for a comprehensive look into this condition. She often cautions against flaring out the lower ribs!

[25] Arthur Lessac and Deborah Kinghorn. *Essential Lessac: Honoring the Familiar in Body, Mind, Spirit.* (RMJ Donald Publishing, 2014), p. 53.

[26] This exercise is from Katy Bowman's *Diastasis Recti* (Propriometrics Press, 2016). I recommend this book for a comprehensive look at diastasis recti with many movement practices to work toward healing it.

[27] To read more about the tonal current, see Arthur Lessac's *The Use and Training of the Human Voice*, 3rd edition (McGraw-Hill, 1996), pp. 122-133.

[28] The Master Teacher Council and Certified Trainers have redefined how we teach the Structural Vowels in light of inclusivity of all English-speaking cultures, which all have differences in how they feel vowels. Although Arthur Lessac originally taught 11 Structural Vowels in American English in his book *The Use and Training of the Human Voice* (McGraw-Hill, 1996), the current trainers of the Lessac Training and Research Institute acknowledge many more possibilities based on the personal uniqueness of the speaker.

[29] Translation found at https://www.gaia.com/article/lokah-samastah-sukhino-bhavantu (January 23, 2018).

[30] Translated by Nicholai Bachman in *The Yoga Sutras Workbook* (Sounds True, 2010).

[31] For more on this particular type of meditation practice, see Sally Kempton. *Meditation for the Love of It: Enjoying Your Own Deepest Experience.* (Sounds True Publishing, 2011), p. 139-40.

[32] You can find this text at https://blog.pachamama.org/send-peace-and-happiness-into-the-world-loving-kindness-meditation or by entering "loving kindness meditation script" into a search engine.

[33] The other six limbs are *asana* (the yoga poses), *pranayama* (breath-control and regulation practices), *pratyahara* (sensory withdrawal to then draw awareness inward), *dharana* (concentration for mental focus), *dhyana* (meditation), and *samadhi* (complete absorption with the Inner Divine resulting in bliss).

[34] Nicholai Bachman. *The Yoga Sutras Workbook.* (Sounds True Publishing, 2010), p. 102.

[35] Deborah Adele. *The Yamas and Niyamas: Exploring Yoga's Ethical Practice.* (On-Word Bound Books LLC, 2009), p. 45.

[36] Nicholai Bachman. *The Yoga Sutras Workbook.* (Sounds True Publishing, 2010), p. 107.

[37] Parker Palmer. *Let Your Life Speak: Listening for the Voice of Vocation.* (Jossey-Bass, 1999), p. 96.

[38] Nicholai Bachman. *The Yoga Sutras Workbook.* (Sounds True Publishing, 2010), p. 120.

[39] Deborah Adele. *The Yamas and Niyamas: Exploring Yoga's Ethical Practice.* (On-Word Bound Books LLC, 2009), p. 107.

[40] Ibid. p. 128.

[41] Nicholai Bachman. *The Yoga Sutras Workbook.* (Sounds True Publishing, 2010), p. 129.

[42] Deborah Adele. *The Yamas and Niyamas: Exploring Yoga's Ethical Practice.* (On-Word Bound Books LLC, 2009), p. 135.

[43] Ibid. p. 142

[44] Ibid. p. 150.

[45] Nicholai Bachman. *The Yoga Sutras Workbook.* (Sounds True Publishing, 2010), p. 132.

[46] Deborah Adele. *The Yamas and Niyamas: Exploring Yoga's Ethical Practice.* (On-Word Bound Books LLC, 2009), p. 154.

[47] Deborah Adele. *The Yamas and Niyamas: Exploring Yoga's Ethical Practice.* (On-Word Bound Books LLC, 2009), p. 165.

[48] Ibid. p. 166.

[49] This is a summary from *The Tree of Yoga,* (Shambhala Classics, 2002), pp. 7-9.

Lightning Source UK Ltd.
Milton Keynes UK
UKHW011908070223
416598UK00005B/768